TOTALLY TONED ARMS

TOTALLY TONED ARMS

Get Michelle Obama Arms in 21 Days

Rylan Duggan, CSCS

WELLNESS CENTRAL

NEW YORK   BOSTON

Copyright © 2010 by Rylan Duggan
Photos copyright © 2010 by Adonis Fitness
All rights reserved. Except as permitted under the U.S. Copyright Act of 1976, no part of this publication may be reproduced, distributed, or transmitted in any form or by any means, or stored in a database or retrieval system, without the prior written permission of the publisher.

Wellness Central
Hachette Book Group
237 Park Avenue
New York, NY 10017

www.HachetteBookGroup.com

Wellness Central is an imprint of Grand Central Publishing.
The Wellness Central name and logo are trademarks of Hachette Book Group, Inc.

Printed in the United States of America

First Edition: January 2010
10 9 8 7 6 5 4 3 2 1

Library of Congress Cataloging-in-Publication Data
  Duggan, Rylan.
  Totally toned arms : get Michelle Obama arms in 21 days / Rylan Duggan.
    —1st ed.   p. cm.
  ISBN: 978-0-446-56335-2
  1. Exercise for women. 2. Arm exercises. I. Title.
  GV508.D84 2010
  613.7'148—dc22   2009035921

This book is dedicated to those who will take the crucial steps beyond simply reading the words contained within these pages, by putting the methods to use. May your results speak for themselves.

CONTENTS

ACKNOWLEDGMENTS

I WOULD LIKE TO EXPRESS my sincere gratitude to a few people who were instrumental in the creation of this book. First of all, thank you to Ashley at Keylight Photography in British Columbia for her fantastic job in translating the exercises into easy-to-follow, step-by-step photographs. Her expertise, professionalism, and attention to detail were crucial in completing this book on time. Second, to all of the staff at Hachette Book Group who have worked on this project and helped bring it to light. There is a tremendous amount of effort that goes into publishing a book, and while the author usually takes the credit, those "in the background" deserve a great deal of that recognition. In particular, I would like to extend my deep appreciation to my editor, Natalie Kaire, as well as Amanda Englander and Leah Tracosas for all of their support, hard work, professionalism, and enthusiasm for this project; I simply could not have done it without them.

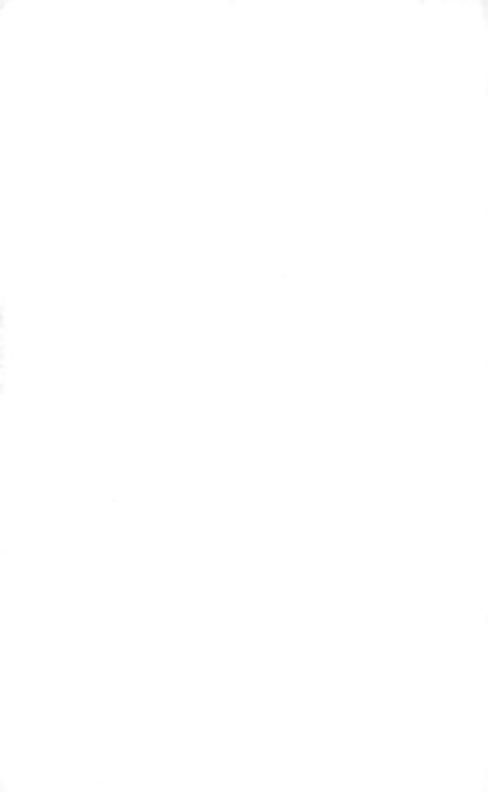

Introduction

The World's First Arm-Toning Expert

When I first got into the fitness industry, I didn't expect that I would eventually become the internationally known authority on women's arms.

As a personal trainer and specialist in women's body sculpting, I always heard countless stories from women about how frustrated they were with their bodies, and more specifically, their arms. They hated the way they flapped and sagged. They yearned for totally toned arms.

This whole "arm problem" was such a common complaint with my clients that I eventually created a website, e-book, and blog specifically to help women conquer this pervasive issue. The program was called Go Sleeveless, and it surprised even me with how successful it became in what seemed like a very short period of time. However, I was not prepared for what was about to happen next.

When President Obama was elected to office, the media frenzy surrounding First Lady Michelle Obama's arms reached startling proportions. People were in awe of how she looked in sleeveless tops, and how sculpted and toned her arms were. As an expert on the subject of women's arms, I started receiving media requests from many sources, including some of the nation's top newspapers, magazines, and even CNN, asking me to give them tips for how their readers could get the coveted "Michelle Obama Arms." This was in addition to the e-mails that began piling up in my in-box from readers of my

Go Sleeveless Blog and e-book. The difference now was that instead of asking me how they could get better arms, they were asking me how they could "get arms like Michelle Obama's."

With a completely packed schedule, a growing wait list of clients, and an e-mail in-box that was on the verge of crashing my hard drive, I decided that the time had come to reveal the program that only my private clients had access to—to the general public. These are the methods that will allow any woman, regardless of age, fitness level, or present condition of her arms, to get "Michelle Obama Arms." This is the program that's worked for countless clients of mine, and I'm confident that it will work for you, too!

Introducing the Totally Toned Arms Program

This book is your one-stop solution to getting toned and sexy arms. No matter how minor or major your problem is right now, the methods I'll teach you in this book will get you the arms you really want.

The program itself consists of a 21-day workout plan, with an additional long-term maintenance system. You will begin with a 7-day quick start routine. For the remainder of the program you will be working out 5 days a week, for approximately 30 minutes each day, following cardio and strength training programs (high-intensity cardio followed by a brief strength training routine). You will be taking weekends off for rest and recovery. You will also follow a simple yet powerful eating plan that works synergistically with both the cardio and strength training programs in this book to bring you even better results.

This program doesn't require you to have a gym membership or use a gym at all if you don't want to. You will be able to do the workout in the middle of your own living room. All you need are a few dumbbells, a resistance band, and an exercise ball to perform every exercise in the program. There are also bonus exercises included for those individuals who prefer to use a gym or have access to more extensive home fitness equipment.

The nutrition program is very realistic and easy to follow. You certainly won't be expected to starve yourself, restrict your calories, or buy any overhyped and overpriced supplements, pills, or shakes. Instead you will eat clean, whole foods, which will stimulate your metabolism, satisfy you, and help detoxify your body, while eliminating foods that cause your body to store fat.

This program will have you working out far less and eating much more than any other fitness and nutrition program you have ever tried—all while delivering even better results.

Sounds too good to be true, doesn't it?

I can assure you it's not, and the benefits of this program don't begin and end with your arms either. By following my three-step method for getting totally toned arms, you will see how this program can literally transform your entire body.

The Three-Step System for Sculpted and Sexy Arms

If you want toned and sexy arms, then my three-step method is the quickest way to make this happen. I have arrived at this process after much trial and error, and I am confident to tell you that by following these guidelines, you will be able to achieve arm-toning results like you never thought possible.

Step 1: Burn the Fat. The most common reason for problem arms is a high body fat percentage. In order for you to have totally toned arms, the number one step is to ensure that you burn off the thick layer of body fat that is covering up the muscles of your arms. Whether you have only a little bit of extra fat, or a whole lot, this is the most important step. Of course, another great benefit of following this step is that you will lose fat not only from your arms, but also from your hips, waist, thighs, and butt. This is where you start to see how the plan will transform your whole body.

Step 2: Sculpt the Muscle. At the same time you are burning body fat, you need to start building and sculpting the underlying muscle. This will ensure that once you have removed the excess fat, the muscle underneath will look its best and will also be firm and toned, giving the skin a solid foundation to form to and eliminating sagging.

Step 3: Boost the Metabolism. To maintain your totally toned arms, then you must increase your metabolism to ensure easy maintenance of your new body. You must increase your metabolism and turn your body into a 24-7 fat-burning furnace. This will allow you to take a break from your healthy eating and exercise program every once in a while and not suffer negative consequences. This also has tremendous benefits for your entire physique. Having a high metabolism keeps your entire body lean, healthy, and energized.

This simple three-step system is your key to success and totally toned arms. By ensuring that all three of these goals are met, your success is inevitable.

The Great Spot-Reducing Lie

Spot reducing is probably the biggest myth ever to plague the fitness world, and sadly, nearly every fitness gadget and gizmo ever sold on an infomercial has been based on this false premise.

If you are unfamiliar with the term, *spot reducing* is the idea that exercising a certain muscle will melt the fat away from that particular spot. For example, doing crunches will give you a six-pack, and squeezing a Thighmaster between your legs will slim down your thighs.

Although this concept has been tested and researched extensively, it has always been proven to be false. What this means is that if you are trying to get rid of fat from a specific area of your body, doing more exercises for that spot is a waste of time. It is true that everybody has a six-pack—the problem is that it's just hidden under a generous layer of body fat. You will never see the toned and sculpted muscle underneath if you do not remove the fat on top, and your arms are no exception.

The Totally Toned Arms Program includes exercises and methods that burn fat from the entire body, and involves a select number of exercises designed to tone and sculpt the muscles of the arms. This is the only true method for getting great arms.

Igniting the Afterburn Effect

The afterburn effect causes a shift in your metabolism and forces your body to burn more fat and more calories when your workout is *over*. Traditional training programs only work *while* you are actually exercising, and that is what makes them so frustrating. That is also why it can seem like you only get results if you are working out for hours a day, every day of the week—you aren't igniting the afterburn effect.

As you follow the program in this book, which takes advantage of this effect, you'll continue to burn calories long after your workout—even in your sleep, for up to 24 hours afterward. Can you see how much of an advantage this can give you in your war against body fat and sagging arms? While other people are spending hours on the treadmill and doing endless exercises—only to have their metabolism shut off the minute they hit the showers—you'll be burning calories and fat long after your workout, and well into the next day.

Here's how the afterburn effect is triggered: When you perform exercises that use large muscle groups, as well as work at high intensity levels for short durations, you turn on hormones that signal your body to burn more calories and melt more fat for the following 12 to 24 hours after your workout. When this is triggered repeatedly, the effect lasts even longer, sometimes up to 48 hours later.

The Three Types of Problem Arms

Most women with problem arms will find their difficulties related to one of the following issues: big arms, sagging arms, or soft arms.

The problem of *big arms* refers to arms that are surrounded by too much body fat. This gives them a much bigger girth and causes that "squishing out" effect you see when you hold your arms close to your sides. This problem almost always coincides with being generally overweight and carrying too much fat throughout the body. Without a doubt, if you have too much body fat on your arms, there are other places on your body where this is true as well.

Many women are afraid of using heavier weights or simply exercising their arms too much because they think their arms will get "too big." This is one of the most prevalent myths that I constantly battle: the fear that women have of "bulking up." However, I have yet to come across a single woman whose big arms were a result of muscle bulk; *in every single case, excess body fat was the problem.*

Women who think they have too much muscle bulk in their arms are often very hesitant to lift heavy weights or do any strength training at all for fear of making their arms even bigger. This is a shame because their fears are entirely unfounded, and it's this mentality that holds them back from real results.

Women cannot build big and bulky muscles, *period.* It is a physiological impossibility. Women do not have the necessary anabolic hormones in their body to build large muscles—namely, large amounts of testosterone and growth hormone. It is true that many female bodybuilders take these hormones in order to bulk up and remain competitive in their sport, but unless you are taking steroids or injections of human growth hormone, you have nothing to worry about.

Building large muscles requires lifting incredibly heavy weights for very few repetitions, eating a tremendous number of calories, and going through long and strenuous workouts consisting of many exercises and multiple sets. Again, you have nothing to fear in this regard. The Totally Toned Arms Program has been carefully designed to avoid each one of these possible conditions. By following the instructions in this book, you need not concern yourself with the possibility of building arms that are big and bulky. If your arms are too big, it's due to *excess body fat* alone. Remove the fat, and your arms will shrink. It really is as simple as that.

Sagging arms are very often a result of weight loss achieved without proper attention paid to toning and strengthening exercises, and in most cases, the faster the weight loss, the worse the sagging. Many women who have successfully achieved substantial weight loss through dieting and reducing calories have found themselves confronted with the unsightly problem of excess loose and sagging skin once they reach their weight loss goal.

This often leads women to believe that their sagging arms are not a result of excess body fat, and in turn causes much frustration and despair as they feel there is nothing left that they can do. However, the reason for the worsening of the sagging skin is directly related to how the weight loss was achieved. As we just discussed, many women who are overly concerned about "bulking up" will often avoid serious strength training exercises and lifting heavy weights.

If they do strength-train at all, they resort to using very light weights and high repetitions. This method of strength training, coupled with a restrictive diet, actually sacrifices muscle mass and will slow down the metabolism. Muscle tissue is then burned up instead of fat tissue, and the end result is actually a *higher body fat percentage* even though the *body weighs less.*

If you fall into this category, don't worry. By following the Totally Toned Arms Program, you can redevelop the lost muscle tissue and begin to burn off the remaining fat and sagging tissue. Your arms will increase their firmness, and the sagginess will reduce. Remember that your skin cells are highly elastic. If a pregnant woman can regain her prepregnancy belly (and indeed she can; I have clients who have achieved six-pack abs after having children), then your arms can bounce back from sagging skin. There is no exception to this rule.

Soft arms is the term I use to describe arms that, although not too big or very saggy, lack firmness, tone, and definition. This is often referred to as the *skinny-fat syndrome.* People who are skinny-fat may seem lean and slim by most standards, and usually have an average body weight, but they actually have a very high percentage of body fat owing to a lack of lean muscle tissue.

The skinny-fat condition is actually very common, but there are certain steps that you can take to prevent or reverse the undesirable consequences of this syndrome. Again, this is often a result of maintaining a low body weight through calorie restriction and dieting that sacrifices muscle tissue, while avoiding exercises and nutritional habits that trigger fat loss.

This also occurs when the exercise program overrelies on cardio and avoids heavy weights and significant strength training exercises. In this case, the muscles literally turn soft, losing any firmness or tone they once had. However, with the Totally Toned Arms Program, you will easily remedy the problem of soft arms and the skinny-fat syndrome by building lean and toned muscle, putting an end to calorie restriction, and ending the long, boring, muscle-wasting cardio sessions you're probably used to.

Now that you have an idea of what this program will do for you, and some of the cutting-edge techniques that we will be using to get you the arms (and the body) of your dreams, let's get started.

First, I'll walk you through the strength training exercises step-by-step. Then, I'll give you an overview of the cardio and nutrition aspects of the Totally Toned Arms Program. Finally, on pages 129–167, I'll provide a daily regimen for 21 days, incorporating all these elements.

Strength Training

ON EACH DAY OF THE Totally Toned Arms Program, you will be given a set of strength training exercises to perform, as well as detailed instructions for how many repetitions and sets to complete and the proper amount of rest time to take between exercises.

The Equipment

This program requires only very basic exercise equipment and does not rely on any specialized machines. The entire workout can be done at home, regardless of available space, but it can also be done at any commercial fitness facility or health club.

I have provided optional "Gym Versions" for many of the exercises in this program, but in any case, you may choose between the "Home Version" or the "Gym Version" at your liking, with no detriment to potential results.

If you are considering upgrading your home gym with more specialized equipment, please have a look at the "Recommended Home Exercise Equipment" section for more information on the exact equipment I used in the making of this program.

The Essentials

▶ Assorted dumbbells (or adjustable dumbbells) from 5 to 25 pounds in 5-pound increments (the actual weights required will vary depending on your individual strength level, but 5 to 25 pounds are suitable for most women)

▶ A stability ball (also called a Swiss ball or exercise ball)

▶ A "medium" resistance band with handles

Optional—For at Home or Gym Use

▶ An exercise bench capable of various degrees of incline

▶ Lat pull-down, chest press, and cable machines

▶ A treadmill or elliptical cardio machine

Note: If you need help identifying the above equipment, please ask the staff at your local fitness facility to point them out to you and give you proper instruction on using their particular style of equipment.

Recommended Home Exercise Equipment

Free Weights

Free weights are essential to any training program, but it's often difficult to know exactly what sizes to get. For the average woman, I recommend getting a set of dumbbells that range from at least 5 to 25 pounds in 5-pound increments. As a general rule of thumb, I recommend getting at least two sizes heavier than 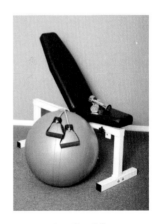 what you could currently use in a chest press exercise for 10 reps.

The dumbbells used in the exercise photos for the Totally Toned Arms Training Program are for demonstration purposes only and should not be taken as an indication for how much weight you should use for the exercise.

Dumbbells can be found with relative ease at garage sales, in classified ads, and even in your friend's basement—it seems everyone has a set of these collecting dust somewhere. And owing to their heavy-duty nature, no matter how "used" their condition is, they should work just fine.

However, if you want to pick up a new set, I recommend visiting your local fitness equipment retailer to find the best deal. Purchasing free weights online can be cost prohibitive because of excessive shipping expenses, unless you can find a company that offers free shipping.

Stability Ball

Stability balls or exercise balls can be found through numerous online retailers or your local fitness equipment store. The ball used in the exercise demonstration photos is a **Fitter First 55cm Classic Exercise Ball Chair** and was selected because of its high durability and resistance to stretching and bursting. Many low-quality fitness balls use an inferior plastic that expands too much and loses its shape during many exercises. These balls often have a shiny and smooth texture, while the higher quality balls have a slightly rough and thick texture. You can find this exercise ball at www.fitter1.com as well as a height chart to help you determine the proper size ball based on your height.

Resistance Bands

The resistance band used in this program is **Professional Exercise Tubing with Handles**, from www.performbetter.com, and is classified as "medium" resistance. Again, it's going to depend on your own personal strength level as to what resistance level you will need, but I usually recommend getting at least one light and one medium band for the average woman.

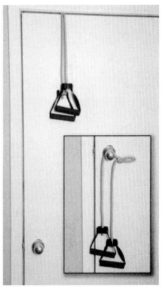

Note: To attach resistance bands to a door, simply tie a knot in the middle, then place the knot on the opposite side of the closed door as shown in the photo at right—and make sure the door is latched securely before exercising. A video demonstration for how to do this properly can be seen on my YouTube channel at www.youtube.com/user/AdonisBHK01—watch the video titled "Using Resistance Bands in Your Home Gym."

At the Gym

Exercise Bench

The exercise bench used in this program is a flat/incline bench that is capable of various degrees of incline all the way up to straight up and down. I recommend using a bench that is sturdy and can easily support your body weight plus an additional 75 to 100 pounds to ensure maximum safety. This is important when performing exercises such as weighted step-ups, when you will be standing on the bench with extra weight. Many benches are built for easy storage, and sacrifice stability as a result. This can lead to tipping over or collapsing during certain exercises. The model I recommend that is best for storage and stability is the **Hoist Flat to Incline Bench**, which can be found at www.hoistfitness.com.

Universal Home Gym

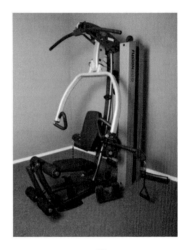

The universal home gym used in this program is the **Fusion 500 by Body Solid**. This gym was selected because of its compact size, solid build quality, and simplicity for home use. This particular model has all the required attachments for the lat pull-down, machine press, and cable exercises demonstrated in the Totally Toned Arms Training Program, as well as a unique feature called Functional Training Arms. These are two cable arms that stick out from the sides of the machine that can be adjusted to any angle for a multitude of cable exercises and replaces the need for resistance bands. You can find this gym at www.bodysolid.com.

Elliptical Cross-Trainer

In the "Cardiovascular Training" section, I recommend elliptical and treadmill machines as the two best exercises for the Totally Toned Arms Training Program (although you will have other options). Between the two, I recommend the elliptical over the treadmill for its superior ability to give a great high-intensity workout, without the added stress on the joints that a treadmill can cause. The elliptical that I use in my personal training studio is an **Endurance E7 HRC**, also from **Body Solid**. I like this machine because of its small footprint, long stride pattern, and very sturdy frame.

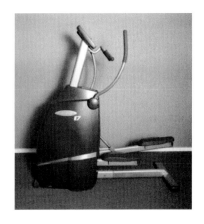

Ellipticals often vary greatly in their stride pattern, and many of the ones I have tested have been too "shallow" to provide a proper workout. The result is that it's harder to get your heart rate high enough, and the movement itself feels much more unnatural. The Endurance E7 HRC defeats both of these problems, and it also comes with its own heart rate monitor and programmable console for supereasy monitoring of your heart rate during interval training. This elliptical machine can be found at www.bodysolid.com.

The Totally Toned Arms Strength Training Philosophy

My training philosophy is "Less Is More." The Totally Toned Arms Strength Training Program will take you less than 15 minutes each day, and you can do it in your own living room.

The key here is that you do not have to sacrifice results for convenience. Most people who exercise for hours do so because they think that that is the only way they can get results, not because they enjoy it. However, when you learn the "Strength Training Secrets" that I will reveal to you in a moment, you will find that an incredibly effective workout can take you literally *minutes a day* while netting you better results than those poor sods sweating away for hours in the gym.

Strength Training Secret 1: Use All Your Muscles

In this program you will notice a preference for exercises that move your entire body. Take, for instance, the sumo squat with shoulder press, weighted step-ups, and jackknife exercises. Each of these exercises works nearly every muscle in your body. You end up killing more than *three birds with one stone*.

For example, the sumo squat with shoulder press replaces all of the following gym exercises:

- ▶ Leg extension
- ▶ Hamstring curl
- ▶ Inner thigh machine
- ▶ Outer thigh machine
- ▶ Shoulder press
- ▶ Hip extension machine

What's more, all these exercises together are still unable to match the results that the sumo squat will. Because this exercise is done free-standing, without the support of a machine, it forces you to work your core (low back and abdominal muscles) to a much greater degree, and all the smaller stabilizing muscles that help you hold your posture.

This one exercise literally replaces more than six others. Can you imagine how much time this will save you?

But that's not where the benefits end. Because you are activating all these muscle groups at once, you stimulate your metabolism to a much greater degree by igniting the afterburn effect, something that will not happen by performing many one-muscle-group exercises.

All of this equates to fewer exercises, higher metabolism, more fat loss, and less time.

Strength Training Secret 2: Lift Heavy Weights

Recall from the Introduction our discussion about the myths of lifting heavy weights. Since you now know that you have nothing to fear by lifting heavy weights, it's time to put them to use. By lifting heavier weights, you increase your exercise intensity to a much greater degree and trigger those fat-burning hormones that ignite the afterburn effect as a result.

You also have to do far fewer sets of a given exercise to get the same, or better, results. This is because increases in muscle strength and tone are triggered by breaking down muscle fibers through lifting weights. For someone who uses light weights, the only way to break down the muscle fiber is by wearing them down over repeated sets, sometimes upwards of 5 or 6 sets for a single exercise. However, if you instead lift a weight that is heavy enough that it causes you temporary failure around 8 to 12 reps, you will achieve this breakdown of the muscle tissue in only 2 or 3 sets.

If that isn't enough to convince you that you need to lift heavier weights, here is another important tidbit of information: You can actually prevent or stop osteoporosis by lifting heavy weights. Heavy weights actually cause the bones to build up their strength to prevent fractures. This is something that doesn't happen with light weights.

By lifting heavy weights and taking every set to temporary failure, you will shorten your workouts, kick-start the afterburn effect, get better results, and build stronger bones.

Strength Training Secret 3: Make It Short and Sweet

If you watch the average gym-goer, they never seem to be in much of a hurry. They might wander around, do a set here and there, chat with a friend, and generally waste time. In an hour, they might complete only two or three exercises.

In the Totally Toned Arms Strength Training Program, you will be performing your exercises in a circuit fashion. This means you transition from one exercise to the next without taking any time to rest in between. You will be resting, but only briefly, at the end of your circuit before repeating it again for the required number of sets.

This type of training keeps your heart rate up, and it keeps your metabolism burning hot. You don't have time to cool off between exercises, making each set highly productive. This style of training also shortens your workouts dramatically. You can literally finish half of your entire workout in the same time that it would take the average person to finish just one exercise.

This type of training also avoids the "cortisol pitfall," as I like to call it. Workouts that last longer than an hour trigger the release of the hormone cortisol. This hormone is needed to combat the rapidly increasing inflammation caused by a long workout. Cortisol is the anti-metabolism hormone: It makes you store body fat, it breaks down muscle tissue, and it's generally counterproductive to getting a toned and sculpted body.

The Totally Toned Arms Strength Training Program is highly efficient, so there will be no hour-long workouts here. No time is wasted, and every *minute* you spend exercising will be getting you results.

Three Steps to Ensure Never-Ending Results

If you've done any reading in health and fitness magazines, you will inevitably hear about the dreaded "plateau." This is the point at which all improvements in your physique seem to come to a complete and abrupt halt even though you continue to stick to your exercise and nutrition program religiously. You may have already experienced this yourself in previous programs you've attempted, and that may even be why you are reading this book now—you are searching for ways to get your body past this sticking point.

The plateau can be one of the most frustrating things about any exercise program, but it's actually quite easy to avoid if you follow a few simple steps from the very beginning.

Step 1: Progressively Overload Your Body

This is probably the simplest way to ensure that your body is always changing and adapting and improving. If during each and every workout you strive to improve even slightly from your last workout, you can be certain that you will continue to burn fat and build lean muscle each and every day. I am still amazed at how many people keep performing the exact same workout day after day, month after month, and wonder why they aren't getting any results.

When you first start a workout, your body isn't used to any of it, so it has to adapt. It adapts by building stronger muscles, and burning up extra body fat to fuel your workout. However, not long after starting a new training program, your body becomes perfectly capable of meeting the demands of the new activity level and has no reason to adapt any further.

Here is where the principle called *progressive overload* comes into play. This principle states that in order to get constant improvements and avoid plateaus, you must continually increase the overall difficulty of your exercise program. This can be achieved through the use of heavier weights, increased numbers of sets and repetitions, less rest time taken between exercises, and other such variables.

The Totally Toned Arms Training Program has progressive overload *built in*. The exercises, sets, and repetitions are structured in such a way that you will automatically be increasing your workout difficulty week by week.

Step 2: Take Each Set to Temporary Failure

Aside from performing the exact same workout each day, this is the next biggest reason why people hit plateaus in their training programs. Many people simply choose a weight that lets them get the minimum number of reps, but never challenge themselves beyond that point.

For example, let's say you are instructed to do 10 repetitions of an arm curl exercise. You select 8-pound dumbbells as a comfortable weight, and do your 10 reps, feeling satisfied that you've accomplished the task at hand. However, if *in actuality*, you could do 15 reps with 8 pounds, then by stopping at 10 reps you haven't even come close to challenging your muscles, and you are far from temporary failure. This would net you zero results.

Here is a critical point: **The number of reps you are instructed to complete in this program assumes that you are taking each and every set to *temporary failure*.** This means that you must use a weight that allows you to achieve the number of reps given, but *not more* and *not less*.

How do you know when you've reached temporary failure? If you cannot complete one more repetition while still keeping proper form—that is temporary failure.

Challenge yourself on *every single set*, and don't stop until you've reached temporary failure. If that means you can actually do 15 reps of an exercise when the program is telling you to do 10, then obviously you will know it's time to increase the weight.

On the other hand, if you chose a weight that is too heavy, you won't be able to get the minimum number of reps, and you will know that a lighter weight is in order.

Note: By taking each set to temporary failure, you will be able to determine the appropriate weights for *you* for each exercise. However, through this process you might find that some of your sets end up going well above or below the prescribed number of repetitions. In this case, you would not count such a set. Adjust the weight, and once you are able to achieve temporary failure within the prescribed number of reps, then count the set toward the total.

Step 3: Constantly Increase Your Cardio Intensities

When beginning a cardio training program, many people stick with the same level or "intensity" for months. Cardio always feels like a challenge at first, but eventually your body adapts and it begins to feel more comfortable with the exercise you have chosen. However, at this point, most folks don't bother to up the speed or difficulty any more than where they started in order to avoid the challenge. This is a notorious results killer.

The Totally Toned Arms Cardio Program will have you doing interval-style cardio training that has you alternating between periods of high intensity and low intensity. You will be judging your intensity level by either "perceived exertion" or by optionally calculating your personal heart rate zones. If you opt to use a heart rate monitor and calculate your intensity levels, this is dead simple. All you need to do is ensure that you achieve the same heart rates week to week, and then you know beyond a shadow of a doubt that your body is being challenged as much on the third week as you were on the first.

However, if you will be going by perceived exertion, this becomes a little more subjective and requires diligence on your part to constantly challenge yourself. You should be making an effort to increase your difficulty level every week or two. It doesn't have to be much, but by making small incremental increases in your speed, level, or intensity, you will ensure constant improvements all the way through the program.

For example, if you chose to use the treadmill, you might increase the speed by 0.2 mph each week. If you are jogging outdoors, you might try and cover an additional block in the same amount of time, or maybe two additional telephone poles. If you are skipping rope, you would try to get an additional 50 to 100 skips in the same amount of time.

The key to constant improvement with your cardio exercise is to *do more work in the same time,* and you will always get great results.

The following exercises make up the strength training component of the Totally Toned Arms Program. Note that a chair can be used in place of an exercise bench in all cases. And remember that the at-home versions of these exercises are just as effective as the gym equivalents.

Strength Training Exercises

Band Dips

1. Attach the midpoint of a resistance band to a high point, such as above a door, or wrap it over a chin-up bar (make sure both sides of the band are of equal length).

2. Stand forward slightly, gripping one handle in each hand, with feet together.

3. Start with your elbows back and up as high as they will go comfortably.

4. Push both of your hands down to your sides to lock your elbows out and complete the rep.

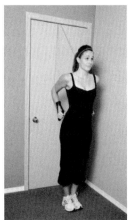 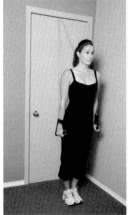

Bench and Ball Dip (Home Version–Dual Chair Dips)

1. Place two chairs facing each other about 3 feet apart.

2. While sitting on one chair, place your heels on the other, and then lift yourself up and just off the edge of your seat (you may have to adjust the distance of the chairs to fit your height).

3. Cross your feet over each other, then bend your elbows to lower yourself down toward the floor as far as you can *comfortably* (the distance you can lower yourself will vary from person to person).

4. Push yourself back up and lock out your elbows to complete the rep.

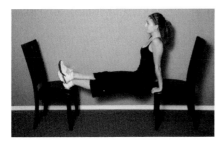

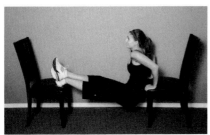

Bench and Ball Dip (Gym Version)

1. Place your feet on a stability ball while sitting on the edge of an exercise bench.

2. Lift yourself up by locking your elbows out and roll ahead slightly so that you clear the edge of the bench.

3. Lower yourself down to the floor as far as possible by bending your elbows, then press yourself back up to lock out your elbows and to complete the rep.

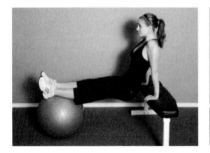 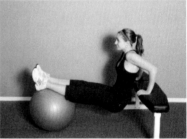

Bench Dips

1. Sitting on a bench place your hands on either side of your hips, and put your feet out in front of you on the floor. Lift yourself up, and just off the edge of the bench to start.

2. Lower yourself down to the floor as far as you can by bending your elbows (if you can't make it all the way to the floor, just go as far as you can and strive to get a little bit lower each time you do this exercise).

3. Push yourself back up to the start position and lock out your elbows (without sitting on the bench) to complete the rep.

NOTE: You can also use a chair for this exercise if you do not have a bench.

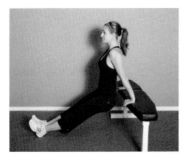 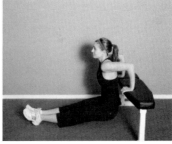

Bench Push-Ups

1. Place your hands slightly wider than shoulder-width apart on an exercise bench (you may also use a countertop or chair), and position your torso over the bench so that your hands are underneath your shoulders.

2. Keep your back straight, and lower your torso down to touch the bench.

3. Push yourself back up, locking out your elbows to complete the rep.

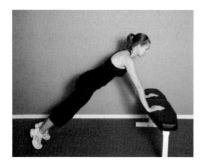 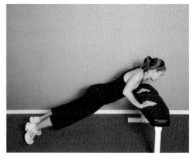

Burpees

1. Stand with your feet shoulder-width apart.

2. Bend your knees and quickly drop down to touch your hands to the floor just in front of you.

3. Quickly thrust both of your feet behind you by hopping up slightly.

4. Reverse the movement by quickly hopping your feet back toward your hands.

5. Stand to complete the rep (this exercise is to be done quickly for best results).

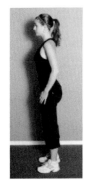 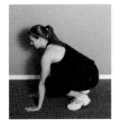 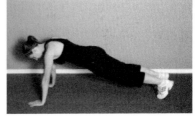

Cable Curl 21s (Home Version)

1. Stand on a resistance band with both sides at equal length.

2. For the first 7 reps, you will curl the handles from bottom to halfway only.

3. After completing 7 reps from bottom to half, pause at the halfway point, then curl all the way to the top. Complete 7 more reps from halfway to top only.

4. After completing these 7 reps, you will then curl full range, from bottom to top, for an additional 7 reps, totaling 21 reps in all.

5. Throughout the exercise, keep your back straight and your elbows tucked into your sides (do not bring your upper arms forward during this exercise).

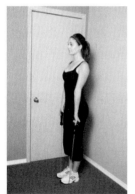 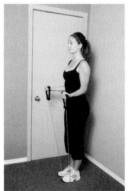 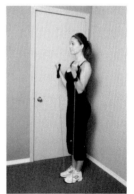

Cable Curl 21s (Gym Version)

1. Using a low cable pulley and a straight bar, stand with your back straight and a palms-up grip with the bar near the midpoint of your thighs.

2. Curl the bar from the bottom to halfway, holding for half a second at the midpoint before lowering back down to the start. Complete 7 reps in this fashion.

3. On the seventh rep, go from halfway to full, and complete 7 more reps from the halfway point to the top.

4. Once you have completed 7 reps in this fashion, complete another 7 reps through full range of motion (all the way from the top to the bottom) to complete a total of 21 reps.

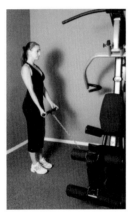 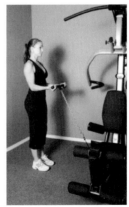 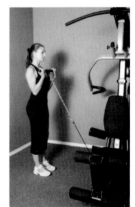

Chest Press (Home Version)

1. Lie on the floor with a dumbbell in each hand, your knees up, and your elbows out to the sides of your shoulders and bent at 90 degrees.

2. Press the dumbbells directly upward and in to touch the ends of the dumbbells together. Hold for a second to squeeze the chest muscles.

3. Slowly lower the dumbbells back down to the starting position to complete the rep.

NOTE: Your upper arms will contact the floor and restrict your downward movement. It is important not to "rest" at this point; you want to keep constant tension on the muscles. As soon as you touch the floor with your elbows, immediately begin the next repetition.

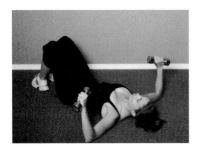 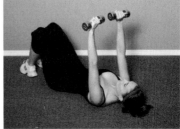

Chest Press (Gym Version)

1. Position yourself with your back straight on a flat chest press machine so that your elbows are positioned out to the side and behind your shoulders.

2. Use a palms-down or palms-in grip, and press the machine arms out to full elbow lockout.

3. Bring your arms back with your elbows behind you to make sure you feel a slight stretch in the shoulders and chest to complete the rep—do not let the weight stack touch down.

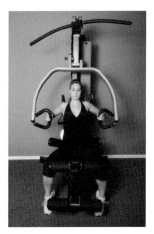 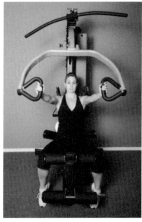

Chin-Grip Pull-Down (Home Version)

1. Attach a single resistance band at its midpoint above a door, so that both sides of the band are of equal length.

2. Stand back from the door with your feet close together and bend forward from your waist to match the angle of the bands.

3. Extend your arms above your head to full elbow lockout for the starting position.

4. Pull the handles down, keeping your palms up, and bring the handles all the way down to the front of your shoulders (keep your elbows close to your sides).

5. Hold here for a second, and then return your arms above your head to complete the rep.

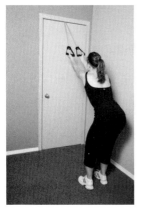 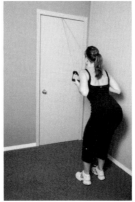

Chin-Grip Pull-Down (Gym Version)

1. On a lat pull-down machine with a long or short bar, grip the bar with your palms up, about 6 inches apart.

2. Lean back slightly, and pull the bar down to the top of your chest, keeping your elbows tucked into your sides.

3. Extend your arms back up to full lockout to complete the rep.

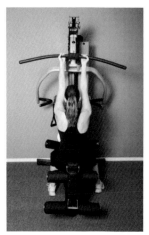 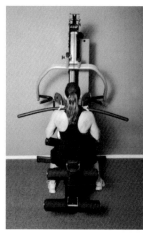

Clean and Jerk

1. Hold two dumbbells at the floor, keeping your back straight and your hips up.

2. In one quick motion, pull the dumbbells from the floor all the way up to the shoulders.

3. As soon as the dumbbells reach your shoulders, squat down slightly for extra momentum, then thrust the dumbbells up into a shoulder press and hold for half a second.

4. Slowly lower the dumbbells back down to your shoulders, then to your thighs, and finally to the floor to complete the rep. This exercise is to be done fast on the way up, using momentum to help you lift the weight, but slow and controlled on the way down.

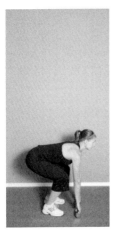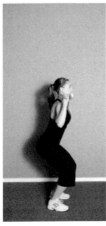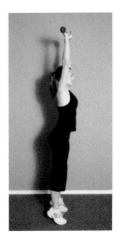

Dumbbell Burpees

1. Hold a dumbbell in each hand by your side, and stand with your feet shoulder-width apart.

2. Quickly squat down and place the dumbbells on the floor (you should still be gripping the dumbbells with your knuckles pointed at the floor) and then thrust your feet behind you into a push-up-like position.

3. Keep your back straight, making sure not to let it droop down, and then quickly hop your feet back toward your hands and stand up to complete the rep.

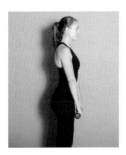
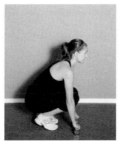

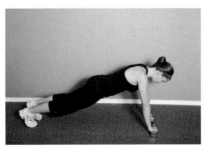

Dumbbell French Press (Bench and Floor Options)

1. Lying on an exercise bench or the floor, hold two dumbbells directly above you with your palms facing each other.

2. Move your arms back to the starting position at a 45-degree angle and hold your upper arms in this position throughout the exercise.

3. Bend your elbows to let your hands drop behind your head, touching the dumbbells to the top of the bench, or just to the floor.

4. Extend your arms back to the top of the movement by locking out your elbows to straighten them. Do not move your arms back to directly above your face; keep them angled backward until you complete the required reps.

BENCH OPTION

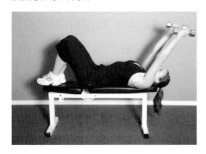 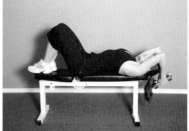

FLOOR OPTION

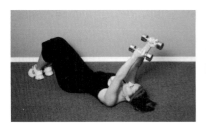 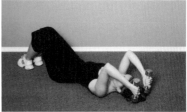

Get-Ups

1. Lie on your back with your legs stretched out and one arm directly above you holding a dumbbell.

2. Keeping the dumbbell directly above you, sit up with the assistance of your opposite arm, while bringing your knees up at the same time.

3. From this position, still keeping the dumbbell positioned directly overhead, stand up with your arm outstretched.

4. Reverse the movement to bring yourself back down to the floor, lying down to complete the rep.

5. Do the required number of reps for one side; then do the same reps for the opposite side to complete the full set.

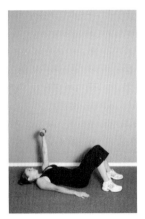 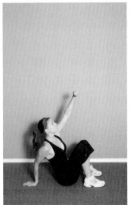 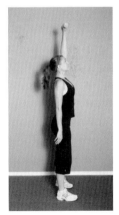

Jackknife

1. Get yourself into a push-up position with your hands on the floor spaced slightly wider than shoulder-width apart, and your shins balanced on a stability ball.

2. Tuck your knees up by rolling the ball toward you as you maintain balance on your hands.

3. Roll the ball back to the start position to complete the rep. Ensure that your back does not droop down and that your hips do not rise up while holding this position.

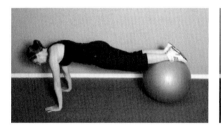 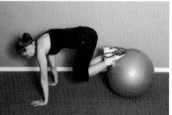

Kneeling Chin-Grip Pull-Down (Home Version)

1. Attach a resistance band above a door with both sides of the band at equal lengths.

2. Kneel on the floor with one knee up, with your front foot about 12 inches away from the door.

3. Lean forward slightly while keeping your back straight and extend your arms in front of you to lock out your elbows in a palms-up grip.

4. Pull the handles down to the front of your shoulders, keeping your elbows close to your sides.

5. Extend your arms back to elbow lockout to complete the rep.

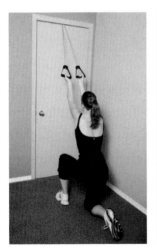 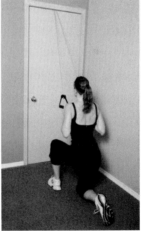

Kneeling Chin-Grip Pull-Down (Gym Version)

1. Kneel on the floor in front of a lat pull-down machine with one knee up.

2. Grasp a straight bar in a palms-up grip with your hands 6 inches apart.

3. Lean forward slightly while keeping your back straight and extend your arms in front of you to lock out your elbows.

4. Pull the bar down to the top of your chest, keeping your elbows tucked in to your sides.

5. Extend your arms back to elbow lockout to complete the rep.

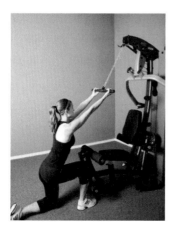 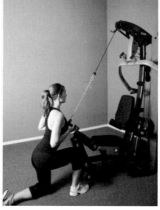

Lat Pull-Down (Home Version)

1. Attach a single resistance band at its midpoint above a door, so that both sides of the band are of equal length.

2. Take a step back and then kneel with one knee down and one knee up.

3. Stretch your arms above your head with your hands shoulder-width apart and palms down.

4. Lean forward from your waist to match the angle of the bands.

5. Pull both handles down and slightly outward toward your shoulders, while squeezing the muscles of your upper back.

6. Extend your arms back to elbow lockout to complete the rep.

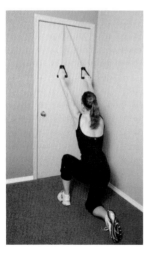 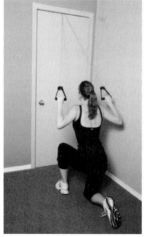

Lat Pull-Down (Gym Version)

1. Using a long bar on a lat pull-down machine, position your hands palms down in a wide grip.

2. Lean back slightly, keeping your back straight, and pull the bar down to the top of your chest, just under your chin.

3. Without leaning forward, extend your arms all the way to full elbow lockout to complete the rep.

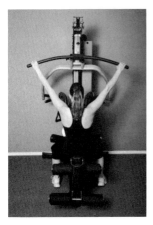 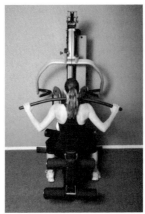

Mountain Climbers

1. Get into a push-up position by placing your hands on the floor, slightly wider than shoulder-width apart.

2. Keep one leg stretched out behind you, and bring your other knee up toward your shoulder with your foot flat on the floor.

3. Start by hopping up and switching the position of your feet as quickly as possible in one quick movement.

4. Repeat this movement in quick succession for the required repetitions. Count one rep for every two switches.

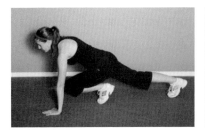 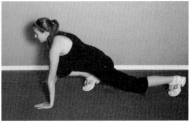

Narrow-Width Dumbbell Press (Bench and Floor Options)

1. Position yourself on a flat exercise bench or on the floor, holding two dumbbells by your chest, no more than 6 inches apart, with your elbows down and by your sides.

2. Push the dumbbells straight up and together, keeping your palms facing inward, and hold for half a second.

3. Lower the dumbbells back down to complete the rep, making sure to keep your elbows tucked in by your rib cage and not up by your shoulders.

BENCH OPTION

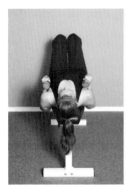 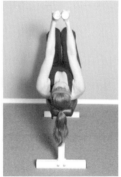

FLOOR OPTION

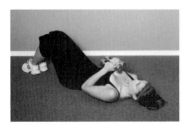 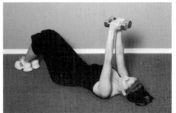

One-Arm Preacher Curl (Home Version)

1. Stand behind a straight back chair, with a dumbbell in your right hand.

2. Place your arm over the back of the chair so that your upper arm is resting against the back.

3. Lean forward to keep your back straight (don't hunch forward), and make sure that your arm is fully extended (if the dumbbell hits the seat before your arm is fully extended, use a chair with a higher seat back, or stand up taller).

4. Curl the dumbbell up as high as possible, without letting your upper arm lose contact with the chair back.

5. Squeeze the bicep for a second, and then lower it back down to complete the rep.

6. Do the required reps on this side; then repeat on the opposite side.

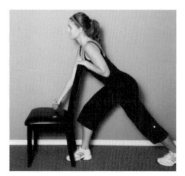 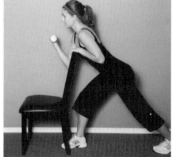

One-Arm Preacher Curl (Gym Version)

1. Position an incline bench into a high incline position (almost vertical) and grasp a single dumbbell in one hand.

2. Position your arm over the back of the bench, keep your back straight, and bend forward far enough so that the top of the bench is positioned under your armpit.

3. Keeping your upper arm touching the back of the bench at all times, curl the weight up until your lower arm is vertical.

4. Slowly lower the weight back down to touch the bench to complete the rep.

5. Repeat the required reps for the opposite side.

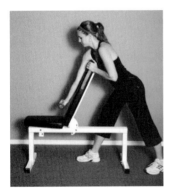 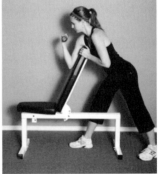

Reverse-Grip Dual-Band Pull-Down and Kickback

1. Attach a resistance band above a door or loop it over a chin-up bar with both sides of the band at equal lengths.

2. Kneel down on one knee and grip each handle with your arms stretched forward and your palms facing up.

3. Lean forward so that your arms are stretched above your head and move back far enough to ensure there is no slack in the resistance band.

4. Start by pulling the handles down toward your chest and driving your elbows back to bring your hands to either side of your shoulders.

5. At this point, keep your palms up and extend your arms back all the way by locking the elbows out. Hold at this position for half a second.

6. Reverse the movement by bringing your forearms forward, then extending your arms back to the starting position to complete the rep.

NOTE: If you can pull the handles down but you can't kick them back, move closer to the band's attachment point to lessen the tension.

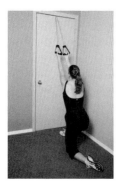 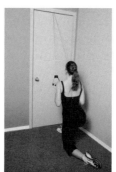 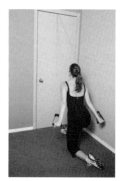

Seated Cable Rotation (Home Version)

1. Sit on the floor with your feet stretched out in front of you and your knees bent slightly.

2. Grasp a single resistance band handle with both hands. The band should be attached under a door, with a knot at about the halfway point to give the proper tension and length.

3. Lock your arms, keep your back straight, and lean back until you feel tension on your abdominal muscles. You should be at the point where you almost fall backward.

4. Keeping your shoulders stationary, and focusing on turning from your waist only, rotate until your hands are just past the midpoint of your torso. Hold here for half a second.

5. Slowly rotate back to the start position to complete the rep. Do the required reps for this side, and then repeat on the opposite side.

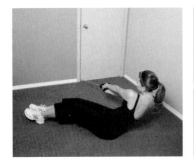
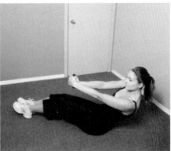

Seated Cable Rotation (Gym Version)

1. Sit on the floor with your feet stretched out in front of you and your knees bent slightly.

2. Grasp a low cable pulley with both hands. The cable should be positioned directly to your side.

3. Lock your arms, keep your back straight, and lean back until you feel tension on your abdominal muscles. You should be at the point where you almost fall backward.

4. Keeping your shoulders stationary, and focusing on turning from your waist only, rotate until your hands are just past the midpoint of your torso. Hold here for half a second.

5. Slowly rotate back to the start position to complete the rep. Do the required reps for this side, and then repeat on the opposite side.

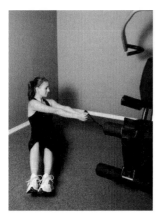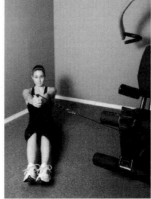

Side-to-Side Push-Ups

1. Place your knees on the ground with your legs together and your feet crossed over behind you.

2. With your hands on the floor together, make sure not to hunch your back up or let your hips droop down.

3. Move one hand out to the side and do a push-up, bringing your torso right down to almost touch the floor.

4. Move your hands back together, then out to the opposite side, and do a push-up on this side as well.

5. Keep alternating left and right to complete the required number of reps for both sides (double the number that is listed).

6. If this exercise feels too easy, then you can do this from your toes instead of your knees.

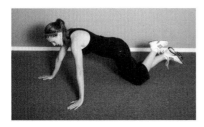
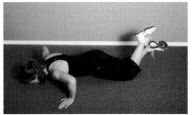
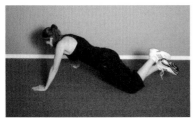
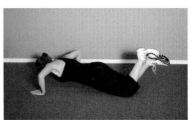

Single-Leg Bench Dips

1. Sit on the edge of an exercise bench with your hands directly by your sides, with your feet out in front of you and bent at 90 degrees.

2. Place one ankle on your opposite leg and lift yourself off the edge of the bench by pushing down with your hands.

3. Lower yourself toward the ground by bending your elbows as much as possible, and making sure to keep your back close to the bench.

4. Push yourself back up to lock out your elbows and complete the rep.

NOTE: You can also use a chair for this exercise if you don't have a bench.

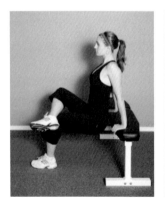 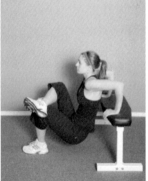

Slow-Down Push-Ups

1. Position yourself in a push-up position, on your toes, with your hands underneath your shoulders and slightly out to the sides.

2. Using control, slowly lower your body down to the floor, taking 4 to 6 seconds to do so (do not just let yourself drop).

3. Once you have reached the floor, get back into push-up position by rocking back onto your knees and assisting yourself up (do not do a push-up to get back to the starting point—you are only slowly lowering yourself in this exercise).

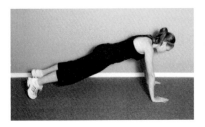 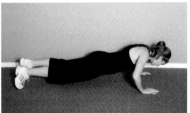

Sumo Squat and Shoulder Press

1. Stand with your feet in a wide stance and your toes pointed out at 45-degree angles, holding a single dumbbell between your palms.

2. Keeping your elbows pointed out to the side and your back straight, squat down to touch your elbows to your knees (or as low as you can get).

3. Stand back up while at the same time pushing the dumbbell directly above you to complete the rep.

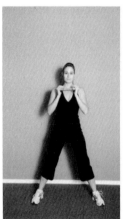 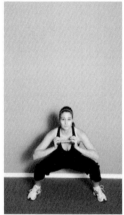 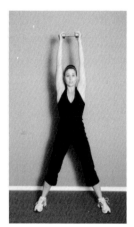

Toe Tappers

1. Position yourself on a stability ball with your hands flat on the floor underneath your shoulders and your shins resting on the stability ball.

2. Take one leg off the ball, extend it as far out to the side as you can, and touch your toe down to the floor for the starting position.

3. Now cross the same leg underneath you as far as you can and touch your toe to the floor.

4. Trying to keep your back as level as possible, continue to move your leg from left to right, touching your toe down to the floor as far apart as possible. One rep is equal to one toe tap on each side.

5. Complete the required reps for this side, and then repeat on the opposite leg.

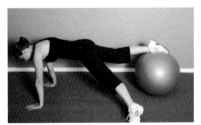 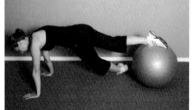

Triceps Push-Downs (Home Version)

1. Attach a resistance band above a door with both sides of the band at equal length.

2. Tuck your elbows into your sides, grip both handles in a palms-down grip, and then stand 2 feet back from the door.

3. Without leaning forward, press the handles down to lock your elbows out (make sure not to pull back with your arms).

4. Squeeze the triceps for a second, and then slowly bring your hands back up to the front of your shoulders to complete the rep.

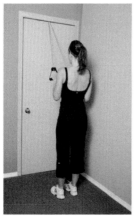 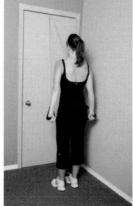

Triceps Push-Downs (Gym Version)

1. Attach a straight bar to a lat pull-down machine, and position your hands palms down and 6 inches apart from each other.

2. Tuck your elbows into your sides, with your hands up by your chest for the starting position.

3. Push the bar down to lock out the elbows, making sure to keep the elbows stationary by your side throughout the movement.

4. Slowly allow the bar to rise back up to the starting point to complete the rep.

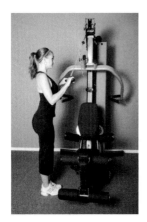 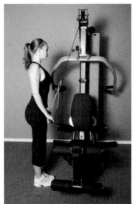

Twisting Single-Arm Pull-Down (Home Version)

1. Attach a resistance band above a door, making sure that both sides of the band are of equal length.

2. Kneel in front of the door, with one knee up and one knee down, with your front foot about 12 inches from the door.

3. With the hand that is on the same side as the knee on the floor, grasp the handle of the resistance band with a palm-down grip, making sure there is no slack in the band.

4. Lean forward slightly and keep your back straight, with your arm fully extended toward the door.

5. Pull the handle down by driving your elbow back and twisting your palm upward as you do so.

6. At the end of the movement, your hand should be by your rib cage with your palm facing up and your elbow behind you.

7. Reverse the movement by extending your arm back to the starting position and twisting your wrist back to a palm-down position to complete the rep.

8. Repeat for the required number of reps using the opposite arm.

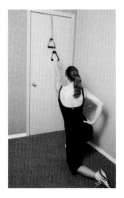 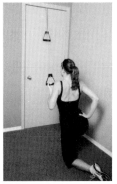

Twisting Single-Arm Pull-Down (Gym Version)

1. Kneel in front of a lat pull-down machine with one knee up and one knee down.

2. Grasp a cable handle from a high cable pulley in one hand, with your palm facing down.

3. Lean forward slightly and keep your back straight with your arm fully extended toward the pulley.

4. Pull the cable down by driving your elbow back and twisting your palm upward as you do so.

5. At the end of the movement, your hand should be by your rib cage with your palm facing up and your elbow behind you.

6. Reverse the movement by extending your arm back to the starting position and twisting your wrist back to a palm-down position to complete the rep.

7. Repeat for the required number of reps on the opposite arm.

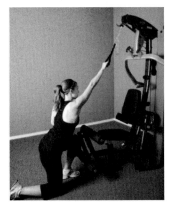 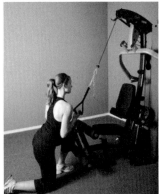

Upward Crunch

1. Position a stability ball under your lower back, with your legs in front of you and bent at about 90 degrees.

2. Lean back over the ball slightly to get a stretch through your abdomen, and hold your arms directly above you holding a single dumbbell between your palms.

3. Push the dumbbell straight up toward the ceiling, holding at the top of the movement to squeeze your abs.

4. Lower yourself back down over the ball, while keeping your arms straight to complete the rep.

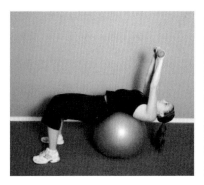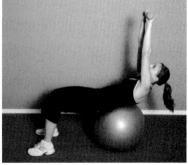

Weighted Step-Ups

1. Hold a dumbbell in each hand and stand with the long side of an exercise bench directly in front of you.

2. Step up onto the bench with one foot, bring your other foot up to meet it, step down with the other foot, and then bring your other foot down to the floor to complete the rep.

3. Step up and down on the bench as fast as possible while maintaining control. One step up and one step down counts as a single rep.

4. For each successive set, start by stepping up with the opposite foot as the set before.

NOTE: If you do not have a bench, you can substitute a set of stairs (usually taking two steps at once to get a similar step height).

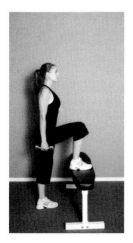 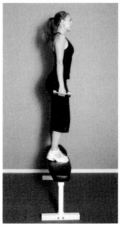

Cardiovascular Training

TRADITIONAL CARDIO AS YOU KNOW IT is dead. I am referring to the type of routine where you pick a cardio machine, set it at one speed, and then go for 20, 30, or more minutes while you listen to your iPod or stare at a TV screen to try and zone out until your time is up.

This type of cardio burns very few calories, does nothing to increase your muscle tone and strength, and certainly does not increase your metabolism. In fact, one 30-minute "traditional" cardio session, for the average woman, will burn less than 180 calories. That is the amount of calories in a *single* sugar-free protein bar! It's simply impossible to lose weight at this rate.

Enter the New Cardio

As I've mentioned, the Totally Toned Arms Cardio Training Program uses a method called *high-intensity interval training,* or HIIT for short. This method of cardio uses very short bursts of high-intensity exercise, followed by low-intensity rest or recovery periods, repeated for a number of intervals.

HIIT is light-years ahead of traditional cardio on all levels. It burns more calories, it ignites your metabolism, it will tone and sculpt your muscles, and it triggers the afterburn effect—the increased calorie burn after your workout—to an incredible degree.

This style of cardio is also much shorter than traditional cardio. In this program, the average session will take you only about 14 minutes! That is less than half the time most people spend on cardio machines at the gym.

It is also very well suited to both beginners and advanced exercisers alike. Because you are only doing very short bursts of high intensity (1 to 3 minutes), even if you are completely out of shape and have never run a mile in your life, you can do this. Advanced exercisers also get the benefit of being able to take their intensity to levels they may not have experienced before, opening up a completely new world of results.

How to Perform a High-Intensity Interval Training Workout

HIIT workouts can be done on pretty much any cardio machine that you would have at home or at a gym, but by no means are you limited to cardio machines. Walking, jogging, swimming, skipping rope, and shadowboxing are all great examples of exercises that work very well in HIIT cardio, and you can even modify some of these to be done in your own living room without ever going outside.

Once you have selected the exercise you will be using, you will then perform a brief warm-up to get your muscles loose and your heart rate up. *Hint*: **A good sign that you are adequately warmed up is that you *just* start to break a sweat.** Immediately after your warm-up, you will start your first high-intensity interval for the time given in your program. For example, you may be asked to go for 3 minutes as hard as you can (see "Knowing How Hard to Work" in this chapter for details on determining your intensity levels). As soon as you have completed the 3 minutes at high intensity, you would then immediately slow down (but *not* stop!) for the time instructed. This will allow your heart rate to drop back down and "recharge" for your next high-intensity interval. The time you take to recover, just like the time for the high-intensity portion, is given very specifically. For example, you may have a recovery interval of only 2 minutes, and immediately after this time has elapsed, you would begin your next high-intensity burst. You would then repeat this cycle of high intensity and low intensity for the number of intervals instructed.

The Totally Toned Arms Cardio Plan

On each of the 21 days in this program, you will begin each workout with your HIIT cardio. This ensures that by the time you begin your strength training exercises, you are well warmed up and your joints and tendons are flexible. Also, the high-intensity intervals will help prepare your muscles for the heavy weights they will be lifting.

Days 1–7: You will be doing a set of three intervals for each of the 7 days, which will consist of 3 minutes high intensity and 3 minutes low intensity.

Days 8–12: You will add one additional interval, while increasing the intensity of your hard interval slightly, and decreasing the duration of both the high and the low intervals to only 2 minutes apiece.

Days 13–14: These will be active rest days and you will not be doing HIIT cardio.

Days 15–19: You will add another interval, making 5 intervals total, while increasing the intensity of the hard interval, and also reducing its duration to 1 minute. Your low-intensity interval will remain 2 minutes long.

Days 20–21: These will be active rest days and you will not be doing HIIT cardio.

Choosing the Best Cardio Exercise

To get the best fat-burning and body-sculpting results, and to ignite the afterburn effect to the greatest degree, you will want to select cardio exercises that involve the entire body.

Recall that strength training exercises that use more, and larger, muscle groups burn more calories and fat. The same holds true for cardiovascular exercise. You want to get your whole body involved to make the most out of the time you spend working out. This means exercises such as recumbent cycling (a stationary cycle with a back rest), stair climbing, and other lower-body-only cardio exercises are poor choices. While these exercises do have their place, they are not well suited to HIIT cardio.

For the Totally Toned Arms Program, the exercise I recommend above all others is the elliptical or cross-trainer machine. This is a machine that mimics a running motion, but also involves upper arm movements (see "The Equipment" section in the "Strength Training" chapter, for a description of the machine I use).

Although the elliptical is very close to a running motion, it does not involve any impact, as your foot never leaves the pedal. This creates easy and fluid motion, involves the entire lower body in a weight-bearing (nonseated) position, and brings the upper body into play with the movement of the arms.

Of course, if you prefer running or jogging and you don't have any joint issues that would make these exercises hazardous for you, then they are excellent choices as well.

For the purposes of the Totally Toned Arms Program, here are the cardiovascular exercises that I recommend in order of preference.

Cardio Exercise Options

Elliptical Cross-Trainer: High-intensity intervals will be achieved using resistance, or "levels," on the machine, plus increases in speed or RPM. You may find that no increases in resistance are necessary, and that increasing your speed alone will allow you to achieve the desired intensity. Recovery intervals will be achieved by reducing speed or resistance.

Walking/Jogging: High-intensity intervals will be achieved either by fast walking, jogging, or sprinting, depending on what it takes for you to get into the proper zone. This can be done outside or on a treadmill. If doing this on a treadmill, you can also use the incline setting to achieve a higher intensity, especially if you are unable to jog or run. Low-intensity intervals are achieved by reducing speed or incline. Jogging in place is *not* an appropriate substitute here.

Rowing: Rowing is a great cardio exercise and can be done on a rowing ergometer, which can be found in most gyms, or of course, on the actual water. High-intensity intervals are achieved by increasing resistance and rowing speed when using an erg, and simply by increasing speed while on the water. Low-intensity intervals are achieved by reducing speed (and resistance when using a rowing erg).

Skipping Rope: Skipping rope intervals are a good option for many because they can be done nearly anywhere. Even if you aren't a good skipper, you can "pseudoskip," whereby you simply do the motion without a rope (handy if you don't have a tall ceiling, or if you tend to trip over the rope a lot). High-intensity intervals are achieved by rapidly increasing the skipping rate, while low-intensity intervals are achieved by slowing the speed. You may also stop skipping during the recovery intervals and simply jog lightly in place instead.

Shadowboxing: This is one of the best cardio exercises to do when you don't have any space or equipment—you don't even need to know how to throw a perfect punch. All you need to do is assume a boxing stance (one foot slightly ahead of the other) and lightly bounce back and forth on the balls of your feet. Keep your elbows tucked in to your sides, and your fists to either side of your jaw. Throw continuous left and right punches, straight forward, for your high-intensity intervals, and then continue the bouncing back and forth motion on the balls of your feet for the recovery intervals. You may also jog lightly in place for the recovery intervals if you prefer.

Swimming: For swimming intervals, lane swimming is best. High-intensity intervals are achieved by increasing your speed using whatever stroke you prefer, and low-intensity intervals are done by slowing your speed down.

Whichever exercise you decide to choose for your cardio sessions, be sure to select one that you are familiar or comfortable with to ensure the best results. While I would suggest that you choose one of the first two exercises based on ease of use, simplicity, and their ability to get consistently good results, any of the above exercises will work well as long as you monitor your intensity levels and keep them in the proper zones, which I will elaborate on next.

Knowing How Hard to Work

Intensity level is something that you have heard me mention a few times already, and that's because it's so pivotal to success in both your strength training and cardiovascular training programs.

While intensity with regards to strength training is usually expressed in terms of how much weight you lift relative to the amount you could lift just a single time (called your 1 rep max), cardiovascular intensity is expressed in terms of percentage of your maximum heart rate.

In the Totally Toned Arms Training Program, you will see that I provide percentage intensities for each of your intervals. For your high-intensity intervals, this will range from 75% to 90%. For your low-intensity intervals, this will be stated as 60% or less.

As an example of how these intensities translate into real-world effort, consider a jogger running down the street: At 0% intensity, he would be standing still. At 50% intensity, he would be walking at a normal pace, at 75% he would be jogging, and his breathing rate would be starting to speed up, and at 100% intensity, he would be sprinting as fast as his legs could carry him, gasping for breath.

Of course, this is all relative to the person exercising. Jogging might be closer to 100% for one person, while it might be only 60% for another. This is why I do not give you actual speeds or levels to work at.

Instead, you will have two options for determining your cardiovascular intensity levels. The first option is to actually calculate your percentage zones with a simple heart rate formula that I will provide you with in a moment. Once you have determined your proper heart rates for each intensity level, you can then use a heart rate monitor while you exercise to help get you into the exact zones.

The second option is to go by perceived exertion, or "feel." It is true that this method is less accurate and more open to error than using heart rates. However, I will show you how to translate percentage intensities into specific feelings of effort, which will help eliminate much of the discrepancy that this method can involve.

Option 1: Calculate Your Approximate Heart Rate Intensities

Use the following formula to find your heart rate (in beats per minute) for each intensity level listed:

▸ Find your max heart rate: 208 – (0.7 × AGE) = _____

▸ Multiply by intensity percentage (i.e., 80%) = _____

▸ Answer = your intensity level in beats per minute

Here is an example for a forty-year-old woman who wants to find her 80% intensity zone:

208 – (0.7 × 40) = 208 – 28 = 180 → 180 × 80% = 144 beats per minute

Fill in your heart rate for each percentage listed below (you may find it helpful to record these numbers on an index card for easy viewing when doing your cardio session).

60%: ____ 65%: ____ 70%: ____ 75%: ____ 80%: ____ 85%: ____ 90%: ____

Use a Heart Rate Monitor for Even Better Results

You could try and take your pulse when you are working out, but it's almost impossible to do unless you come to a complete stop. Furthermore, when doing HIIT cardio, as you are alternating between high and low intensities relatively quickly, there simply isn't enough time to stop and try and find your heart rate before the interval elapses.

This is where a heart rate monitor becomes an invaluable tool. A heart rate monitor is a small chest strap that you wear around your rib cage against your skin. It picks up the electrical activity of your heart and sends a signal to a receiver that you wear on your wrist like a watch. This will tell you exactly what your heart rate is. The best thing is, there is no delay; it tells you instantly what intensity level you are at. You can then use the intensity percentages that you calculated in the previous section to fine-tune your cardio program.

But why is this important? It's quite simple: By using a heart rate monitor, *you can't cheat*. It will tell you when you are working hard enough and if you are hitting your proper intensity zone, and it will also tell you if you are slacking. While "going by feel" and using your perceived exertion level is adequate for the purposes of this program, this can lend itself to a certain amount of error. You may *feel* that you are working harder than you actually are. This is why using a heart rate monitor can get you even better results—if you aren't working hard enough, it will tell you. Conversely, if you are working *too hard*, it will tell you that, too, so you can slow down and avoid premature fatigue. So if you are serious about taking your results to the next level, then you might want to consider picking yourself up a heart rate monitor. Some cardio machines have heart rate monitors built in to track this for you.

Option 2: Ratings of Perceived Exertion

If you do not have a heart rate monitor to keep track of your intensity levels while exercising, then you can also go by feel using your level of perceived exertion. While this is somewhat subjective, by using the guidelines below, you should be able to get an idea of what each intensity zone should feel like while you are in it. It is a good idea to write these levels on an index card for easy viewing during your workout to ensure you are hitting the proper zones.

60%—**Easy:** Can carry on a conversation with no change in breathing

65%—**Light:** Breathing rate increasing, but no problem talking

70%—Average: Feels like a workout, but not too strenuous; can still talk

75%—Moderate: Talking to someone is uncomfortable

80%—Heavy: Can talk in only short bursts

85%—Hard: Unable to carry on a conversation at all

90%—Very hard: Cannot maintain this for longer than 1 minute

95%—Very, very hard: Cannot maintain this for more than 15 seconds

100%—Absolute maximum: Gasping for breath

The Nutrition Program

YOU PROBABLY PICKED this book up expecting to find a detailed workout program that would take you step by step to your goal of getting totally toned arms. And while that is indeed the intention of this program, the workout *alone* is not enough to accomplish the task of transforming your arms.

The importance of proper nutrition—whether the goal is better health, weight loss, body sculpting, muscle building, sports performance, or any other health and fitness goal you may have—cannot be understated, and this program is no exception.

In many cases, nutrition could be the *most important* aspect of your quest to get sculpted and sexy arms, more so than even strength and cardiovascular training. Nutrition can literally make or break your success.

So, if you're one of those people who think that you can offset the effects of a bad diet by exercising, think again. This fallacy will only serve to frustrate you, and keep you locked in a continuous struggle to gain control over your physique.

The program in this book is based on a few basic core principles. If you ensure that your daily eating habits revolve around these principles, then you cannot help but achieve success.

Stick to the guidelines that follow, and you will be able to achieve results that you never thought possible.

The Three Core Principles of Nutrition

Principle 1: Eat Only Clean, Whole Foods

Sadly, many of the foods people eat today are far removed from their natural, healthy form. This overprocessed and packaged food is stuffed full of preservatives and chemicals to make it shelf-stable and convenient for you to pop in the microwave.

These types of foods are a disaster for your health, your body, and your arms in particular. They create toxic buildup in your system (more on that later) and they render you incapable of losing any body fat. They also provide little in the way of nourishment and adequate vitamins and minerals, which are so essential to a well-functioning body.

It's time to turn this around and start eating foods in their natural, wholesome form again. So what exactly does this mean? Well, for starters, you will be doing away with anything that you can't pronounce. What I mean by that is, if you read the food label and in the ingredients list you see something that looks like "titanium dioxide" or "hydrolyzed yeast extract" or "monosodium glutamate," then it's best that you don't eat it.

When you do your grocery shopping, you will find yourself sticking to the "perimeter," where you find the deli, bakery, dairy, and produce sections. Why is this important? If a food is perishable, then it contains far fewer chemicals and preservatives and has more nutrition left intact.

You will be avoiding sugars and high fructose corn syrup. You will be selecting whole grain options such as brown rice, sprouted grain breads, and quinoa as opposed to their highly processed counterparts. You will drink herbal teas and pure water instead of diet sodas and lattes. You will eat servings of lean and unprocessed meats such as turkey and chicken breast, as opposed to highly salted and processed meats such as bacon and salami. You will consume far more fresh fruits and vegetables, and far fewer snack foods such as granola bars and cookies.

By making these changes, you will be able to fuel yourself for your workouts and provide yourself with energy to spare. You will kick-start your metabolism and start burning away extra body fat. You will also provide proper nutrition to improve your overall health, and start seeing other benefits such as improved skin tone and elasticity, and even better hair and nails. You will begin to detoxify and naturally transform your entire body, not only your arms.

Principle 2: Increase Your Metabolism Through Your Diet

Having a high-revving metabolism is key to lasting weight loss and getting a lean, toned, and sculpted body. Exercise is one method to boosting your metabolism, but dietary modifications can help out substantially, as well.

By making changes to your nutritional habits, you can capitalize on many little "boosts" you can give your fat-burning furnace, which, when combined, create a very dramatic overall effect. You can literally revamp your entire metabolism in a matter of 21 days.

You will replace empty calories with calories that will fuel your workouts. Next, you will choose foods that burn more calories. For instance, lean protein requires a significant number of calories to break down, so by including a small portion of lean protein with every meal, you can get multiple metabolism spikes throughout the day. The same is true for high-fiber foods, which include most fruits and vegetables.

You will switch from eating three big meals to having six smaller meals per day. This will balance your blood sugar, reduce fat-storing hormones, and increase the calories you burn—a result of your digestive system working steadily throughout the day.

Principle 3: Detoxify Your Body to Trigger Fat Loss

Most people think of body fat as simply stored energy. And while it's true that body fat is one of the best methods your body has for storing extra energy until it's needed, it also has other purposes.

A less-known function of body fat is to protect you from harmful toxins and waste products. You might wonder what this has to do with getting totally toned arms. Let me put it to you like this: If your body is in an overtoxic state, you will not be able to get rid of your extra fat stores. This is because a toxic body loves body fat.

Few would disagree that the lifestyles we lead can be exceedingly toxic. We work long hours and get little sleep. We drink too much alcohol and caffeine and we breathe in too much pollution. We stress out far too much, and we don't take enough time for rest and relaxation. We spend our days sitting at a desk, and we get far too little exercise. To top it off, our diet is one of the major contributing factors to the toxic load we place on our bodies. The amount of sugar, salt, and preservatives we put in our bodies on a daily basis is staggering. This all creates a very toxic and acidic environment in our bodies.

And while our bodies are incredibly efficient at processing and removing many of these toxic substances, they can only take so much. At some point, the amount of garbage we put into our system exceeds our body's ability to remove it. This is where your fat cells come into play: If your body cannot remove all the toxic waste and by-products that it is receiving, it will stuff them away into your fat cells until such a time that it can deal with them and get them out.

Unfortunately, most people never give their body this opportunity, and as a result, their fat cells continue to grow and expand year after year. This is exactly why some people can exercise a lot, and eat so little, yet *still* not lose any weight. Their body needs the extra fat to protect it from all the toxic buildup. However, if, and when, they allow their body to detoxify and cleanse itself, there will no longer be a reason to hold on to the extra body fat. At this point, weight loss becomes easy and even effortless.

Is Cleansing the Cure?

If you need to detoxify your body to lose weight, then you might think that going on a "cleanse" or a "flush" would be the best course of action. In reality, it's not. *Detox* is a pretty big buzzword these days. There are countless programs, products, and services designed to help you flush your body of all toxic waste in as little as a single weekend. They come with claims of quick and effortless fat loss, better skin and hair, improved regularity, and even elimination of allergies, sinus problems, and many other health issues. But all this is actually overkill, and can even do you more harm than good.

When you take a supplement, herb, or product designed to flush your body out, you cause a cascade of toxic waste to enter your system. While this might seem like a good idea to try and purge everything simultaneously, your body simply can't handle this much at once. The kidneys, liver, and colon are likely a little sluggish to begin with from years of improper eating and an unhealthy lifestyle—which is actually one of the reasons that toxins begin to accumulate in your body in the first place.

Therefore, when you try and force your body to detox all at the same time, it's like trying to continuously flush a clogged toilet—eventually it's going to overflow. In your body, these toxins just recirculate through your bloodstream and make you feel very ill. Many people who go on a weekend cleanse are hit with the harsh reality of just how painful an event this can be. And at the end of it all, you haven't even put a dent in the amount of toxins that your body has accumulated over the years.

How to Detox Naturally

Thankfully, there is an easier and more effective way to detox than by taking a supplement or using a cleansing kit to speed the process, and here it is: The key to safe and easy detox is simply *to stop the further addition of toxic substances into your body*, and then let your body detoxify naturally and safely *on its own*.

It is essential to note that you are constantly detoxifying each and every day, with every breath you take. The key is to stop loading your body up with toxins, and then let your body naturally eliminate whatever it's accumulated over the years. There is no need to force or rush this process; it will happen if you let it.

You can help this process along by following a few specific guidelines. For example, by ensuring that you are eating adequate fiber and drinking enough water, you will be able to improve the rate at which you flush toxins from your body, without any nasty side effects or feeling ill. By following the "Ten Nutritional Commandments," you can rest assured that you will be setting your body up for the natural and safe detoxification that is essential in fat elimination and weight loss.

The Ten Nutritional Commandments

1. Eat Six Smaller Meals a Day

Many North Americans stick to the "three squares a day" rule of breakfast, lunch, and dinner. And while this isn't entirely accurate because many people snack all day long, they still tend to consume the vast majority of their calories in three larger meals. They also tend to eat in an *increasing* fashion: they eat an average breakfast, then a larger lunch, and an even larger dinner.

This business of eating three squares a day, and eating more calories as the day progresses, is an absolute nightmare for fat loss. If you wait too long between meals, your blood sugar drops very low. When this happens, hormones are released that trigger extreme hunger and ravenous cravings. At this point, it will then be all you can do to stop yourself from gorging on the first thing you can find (which is usually something quick and easy from the nearest vending machine). Willpower does not stand a chance against this powerful biological drive to eat.

However, if you eat smaller meals, and eat more frequently, you never let yourself get too hungry, and you balance out your blood sugar levels. You won't ever get to the point where you are ravenous, and you will have a steady stream of energy all day long. Also, you won't get those horrible energy crashes that are so common after large meals.

And finally, because you will be fueling yourself in smaller amounts all day long, your metabolic furnace will be burning up even more calories and fat than you would otherwise. This "hot furnace effect" happens because every time you eat something, your body has to burn calories just to digest what you've eaten. This means that if you are eating constantly throughout the day, your body is steadily using up energy to fuel your digestive processes.

Eating six smaller meals, spaced evenly throughout your waking hours, will result in a much greater calorie burn, a higher metabolism, subdued hunger and cravings, and improved energy levels.

2. Eat Vegetables with Every Meal

I know, I know, you *know* you should eat more veggies. For decades, mothers around the world have been lecturing, coercing, forcing, and begging their children to eat their vegetables. Guess what? You should listen to your mother!

Vegetables are loaded with essential vitamins and minerals and all-around excellent nutrition, yet they are sparse in calories. Compare this to junk foods, which are loaded with calories, sugar, saturated and trans fats, and other harmful substances, but lack real nutritional value.

Today, it is not uncommon to be *malnourished* while at the same time *morbidly obese*. This is because the foods that many people eat are so overprocessed and devoid of any nutritional goodness that they are not getting the bare minimum of essential nutrients their bodies require. At the same time, these foods are so crammed with calories that they provide far more than the human body actually needs. Thus some people continue to gain weight while their bodies suffer the consequences of an inadequate intake of essential nutrients. And because they still aren't getting the nutrients they require, they never feel satisfied and they continue eating. Instead, if they just ate more nutritious foods, of which vegetables may be the most nutritious, they would find themselves much more satisfied and their hunger would go away.

Vegetables play a very important part in the body's natural detoxification process, as well, and can help facilitate fat loss through this method quite effectively. This is partly due to their high fiber content, as well as the phytonutrients that support healthy cell function.

Phytonutrients are what give fruits and veggies their taste, smell, and vibrant color. You've probably heard that you want to have as many colors on your plate as possible (as long as they are natural colors) and that is truly good advice. To put it in the simplest terms, the risk of every chronic disease imaginable, such as heart disease, cancer, diabetes, liver failure, and more, can be reduced by consuming a diet high in fresh vegetables. They support the immune system, increase your energy, detoxify your cells, alkalize your body, and much more.

But veggies for breakfast?

When I tell my clients they need to be eating vegetables for breakfast, I often get skeptical looks. It seems strange to most people to eat veggies for breakfast, especially when they are used to cereals, bagels, and muffins. But this isn't really that out of the ordinary when you think of how many popular breakfast dishes actually contain veggies. For example, you can easily get a whole serving of veggies at breakfast by adding some peppers, tomatoes, and onions to an omelet. Use your imagination and try to get as many veggies as you can, wherever you can. It's nearly impossible to go overboard with them, so eat up.

Juicing is a great way to get plenty of veggies whenever you need them, especially at breakfast. There are even many incredibly healthy organic veggie juices that come prebottled and ready to go so you are never more than a few seconds away from a full serving of vegetables at any time of the day.

3. Eat Fruit with the Day's First Three Meals

The importance of fruit in your nutrition plan follows along many of the same lines as eating adequate vegetables. Generally speaking, fruit contains plenty of fiber to help out your natural detoxification process, along with very high levels of vitamins and minerals, and phytonutrients. The brilliant natural color of many fruits gives hints to the powerhouses of nutrition that they are.

However, there seems to be an ongoing debate as to whether fruit is a good idea when you are trying to lose body fat. This is a result of the fact that fruits contain sugar. While fruit does contain sugar, it is not the same *type* of sugar as what you would find in candy or sweets. The difference is that fruit sugars burn more slowly—which is also known as having a low glycemic index. The fiber content in fruit slows this process down even further, thus avoiding the rapid spike in blood sugar, and therefore insulin, that is so common with most other sweet foods.

However, you will notice that I am instructing you to eat fruit only in each of your three morning meals. By eating fruit at the beginning of the day, it will give you that kick-start of energy you need to get you going in the morning and into the afternoon, but you will also be able to burn off the sugar throughout the day. By noon you should have consumed the vast majority of your daily carbohydrates and calories, and therefore by eliminating fruit from the last three meals of the day, you will ensure that you don't go overboard with sugar.

4. Eat Lean Protein with Every Meal

When it comes to eating for fat loss, lean protein is essential. I say *lean protein* because many protein sources also contain very high amounts of saturated fats and are not well suited to fat loss (e.g., high-fat cuts of red meat, pork, and dark poultry meat). However, lean protein sources, some of which include chicken and turkey breast, lean cuts of beef and pork, tuna, white fish, etc., are all excellent choices. Gram for gram, protein requires the most energy from your body to be broken down and metabolized—it has a very high energy cost. This means that the more lean protein you eat, the more energy your body is going to burn up.

Another great property of protein is its preference to be used as a building block rather than an energy source. While all foods can be converted to body fat when there is an excess, protein is the least likely to do so. Your body much prefers to use protein to rebuild and repair, especially after a hard workout, rather than be stored as fat. This means that if your diet is high in protein, you will burn far more calories than someone eating a low-protein diet. Also, if you do end up eating a few more calories than you intended, and those calories come from protein, then that extra protein is much more likely to go toward repairing your body from your workouts.

And finally, when you consume protein with a meal that also contains carbohydrate, the protein actually slows the rate at which the carbohydrate is converted to blood sugar. And since a quick spike in blood sugar promotes fat gain, by including a little protein with each meal, you can drastically reduce this risk.

For all these reasons, it is essential that you make sure each time you eat a meal, it contains at least a small serving of protein.

5. Eat Only Slow-Burning Complex Carbohydrates

By now, you might feel that carbohydrates are the enemy. Considering that sugar (which is a carbohydrate) spikes your blood sugar, promotes the release of insulin, and causes fat storage, you might think that the whole no-carb movement has some value.

However, I totally disagree with the no-carb philosophy. Carbohydrates do have their place; it's just that most people go *overboard* with them. When you don't eat enough carbs, you slip into a state called ketosis, which can be very hard on your body. You get severe "brain fog" and confusion because your brain needs carbohydrates to function properly. You also become lethargic and your energy is sapped. Getting in an effective workout while you are in ketosis is next to impossible. No-carb diets are very often high in saturated and trans fats, and low in essential vitamins and minerals. They also produce a significant "acid load" on the body, which becomes toxic, and as you now know, this makes it impossible to achieve any sort of weight loss.

Carbs are necessary if you want to exercise efficiently, and they are even needed to trigger fat burning. There is a saying that "fat burns in the flame of carbohydrate," which means that if you don't have any carbohydrates in your system, then you can't burn body fat. In fact, the reason why most no-carb diets work in the beginning is because you have to eliminate many of the foods you routinely eat in excess, and as a result, your total caloric intake drops so low that you lose weight. These diets also massively reduce the amount of insulin your body is secreting because you won't be eating any sugar. However, these effects are short-lived: Your metabolism will soon slow down due to the under-consumption of calories. And because physical activity in the complete absence of carbohydrates is profoundly difficult, your workouts will be dismal, as well. However, the main reason no-carb diets don't work is because they are nearly impossible to maintain long term. You can only eat so much concentrated protein and fat before your body takes over and compels you to eat something with carbs in it. It might take two weeks, or it might be two months, but when this happens, all the weight you lost will come piling back on with a vengeance.

Not all carbs are bad, and if you make appropriate selections, eating carbs can actually help you burn body fat. The key is to avoid carbohydrates that are overly processed and that have a high glycemic index. These include dense starches such as white rice and flour products such as breads, wraps, and many corn products. Also, carbohydrates known as "simple sugars"—such as corn syrup, table sugar, and honey—should be eliminated. These carbohydrates rapidly spike your blood sugar level, leading to excess insulin output, which, in turn, stores body fat.

By replacing these foods with slow-burning "complex carbs," such as fruits and vegetables, and whole-grain and fiber-dense starches, such as brown rice, sprouted grain breads, and sweet potatoes, you will make huge improvements in your levels of energy and your ability to lose body fat. These foods burn slowly, keep energy levels up, provide plenty of nutrition, and balance your blood sugar levels.

6. Don't Restrict Calories–Replace Them

The first thing that most people do when they want to lose weight is to massively reduce the number of calories they eat. As we have already discussed, this is murder to your metabolism. While there is always some initial weight loss, it is short-lived and the overall effect ends up reversing itself when the extra weight is gained back—and then some—from the reduction in metabolism.

If you want to train your body to let go of its extra body fat, you simply cannot restrict your calories. Your blood sugar will drop too low, and you will be plagued by uncontrollable urges to eat everything in sight (especially sweet and fatty foods, which are more calorie dense). Your metabolism will slow down, and your energy levels will suffer, making it impossible to get through an effective workout.

The Totally Toned Arms Nutrition Plan is not about cutting calories and starving yourself; it's about replacing the "bad" foods in your diet with "good" ones. Just by changing the foods you eat, you will find that you aren't consuming nearly as many calories. This is because you will be eating foods that are more nutrient dense, but calorie sparse. You will feel satisfied and full, while at the same time you will increase your metabolism and improve your energy levels.

For example, instead of starting your day with a vanilla latte and a muffin, you might replace that with a fruit smoothie containing fresh berries, low-fat protein powder, and a scoop of powdered greens. This would keep you fuller longer, provide plenty of vitamins and minerals, taste great, and give you energy to spare without the crash afterward.

7. Drink Ten to Twelve Glasses of Water a Day

I know you've heard this before, but it simply cannot be overstated. You need to drink more water. The rule of eight glasses per day is an absolute *minimum* for optimal functioning, and I am recommending ten to twelve. You might be thinking that you don't drink nearly that much water right now, and you haven't had any problems. However, it's important to clarify something here that really throws people for a loop. We've always been told we need eight to ten glasses of water per day, but most people don't get anywhere close to that much. And yet, we don't have people dropping over dead from dehydration all over the place, do we? And we often don't feel very thirsty; otherwise we'd drink more water, wouldn't we? So is this number just some concoction or marketing ploy by the bottled water companies to get you to drink more water? Thankfully, no.

Our bodies are incredibly adaptable, and if you do not provide your body with enough water, it has many mechanisms that prevent dehydration from causing serious problems. First of all, it stops eliminating it. While a normal healthy person can easily eliminate up to 2.5 liters of water per day (10 cups) through urine alone, and at least another liter or more from sweat and feces, in someone who is dehydrated, these processes slow down considerably. This is why someone who isn't drinking enough water can easily become constipated, stop sweating (which throws off the body's temperature-regulating mechanisms), and stop urinating. Interestingly enough, all three of these processes are *major contributors to your natural detoxification mechanisms.*

So if you are not getting enough water, it's easy to see that you are literally putting a grinding halt to your ability to eliminate toxins. Your body will be forced to retain the water that it has, and recirculate it through the body. Think of a creek bed that stops flowing in the heat of summer. The water becomes stagnant, dirty, and scummy, bugs start to show up, and it starts to smell. If you aren't providing your body with enough water to keep everything flowing and moving out, then this is exactly what can happen inside you.

When you get enough water, your body will function optimally. It won't have to retain any excess fluid, and you will notice that you look leaner and slimmer because of it. You will be able to flush out toxins much faster, you will think clearer, your vision will be better, you will have more energy, and the list goes on. Most people don't think they are feeling all that bad until they start drinking more water and realize the difference it makes to their well-being. So drink up!

8. Eliminate Sugar and Artificial Sweeteners Completely

Sugar is to fat loss as kryptonite is to Superman: totally crippling. You cannot eat a diet that contains large amounts of sugar and lose body fat, period.

As I've touched on briefly already, sugar promotes the release of the hormone insulin, and insulin promotes rapid storage of body fat. When insulin is released, it often "overshoots" the amount needed and subsequently causes a sugar crash by the rapid depletion of blood sugar. This causes hypoglycemia, which can cause powerful sugar and carbohydrate cravings, ravenous hunger, confusion, irritability, lethargy, etc.

At this point, the physiological drive to eat becomes so overpowering, you will often find yourself gorging on something that will satisfy those cravings fast. Carbohydrate-laden foods such as bagels, muffins, chocolate bars, etc., get your blood sugar up rapidly, but they will lead to yet another crash and a continuation of this cycle.

This scenario might sound familiar: You start your day with a coffee and a muffin, only to be hungry again and craving something sweet by 10:00 a.m. You then have another cup of coffee, and maybe something from the vending machine to tide you over until lunch. Lunch rolls around and you are starving, so you grab a sandwich and instead of the salad, you opt for the fries because vegetables just won't fill you up enough. The crash hits around 3:00 p.m. and it takes everything you've got not to fall asleep at your desk. You grab another coffee and some chocolate to give you that jolt to help you make it through the rest of your workday with some sort of productiveness. Finally, you head for home, ravenous, tired, and grumpy from a long day at work. You don't have the energy to cook, so you grab a pizza on the way home and quickly dive into a few slices as soon as you get through the door. You then crash on the couch afterward (there is no sense trying to do anything on a full belly) to watch a bit of TV, relax, and recharge. Later you muster enough energy to do a few chores around the house before getting ready for bed. If you are up late, you'll grab another snack sometime around 9 or 10 p.m., which will probably consist of another slice of pizza, and then off to bed you go.

In working with so many clients, I've seen this pattern emerge time and time again. And while the specific foods you eat might be different, my bet is you can probably see a number of similarities between this scenario and your own personal eating habits.

This example illustrates well the "sugar roller coaster." You eat sugar, which causes a crash and makes you crave more sugar. You then eat even more sugar to deal with the cravings, and the cycle perpetuates. This is exactly why obesity rates are skyrocketing and Type II diabetes is reaching epidemic levels. In the scenario I just described, you would have insulin surging through your system all day long, storing up body fat like crazy. You'll also be too tired and lethargic to even think about working out or exercising at all. For these reasons, it's easy to see why sugar is a food that makes you fat, and why it must be avoided at all costs. This includes table sugar, honey, high fructose corn syrup, fruit juices (even natural fruit juice), and fructose. Fruit, when eaten whole, does not apply here.

Also, I highly recommend you eliminate artificial sweeteners such as sucralose (Splenda) and aspartame (Equal). While these foods (or chemicals, I should say) don't affect blood sugar and contain no calories, they are quite acidic and toxic to the body. They also perpetuate sugar addictions, owing to their highly sweet nature, and make it incredibly hard to kick your sugar habit. Also, a frightening number of scientific studies on these man-made chemical sweeteners point to numerous health risks associated with their use.

If you absolutely must use something as a sweetener, I recommend stevia, which is a natural herbal extract that is perfectly safe and won't negatively affect fat loss.

9. Don't Drink Your Calories, and Forget About "Diet" Drinks

Recall Commandment 1 and how eating frequently throughout the day can help you burn calories at an accelerated rate. Remember that each time you eat something, your body burns energy just to digest it. Well, this *does not* happen when you drink something. Because liquids do not need to be mechanically broken down by your digestive system, they don't cause you to burn any additional calories. If you want to boost your metabolism, you simply cannot afford to be consuming liquid calories that aren't going to further you along in your body-transforming goals.

Additionally, since diet drinks contain artificial sweeteners and other chemicals that can potentially add to your body's overall toxic load, you should not be drinking them either (see the previous commandment for more information on the dangers of artificial sweeteners).

As a general rule of thumb, the only beverages you should be drinking are pure water and herbal teas. If you must drink black tea or coffee, then limit yourself to *no more than two cups per day* (caffeine is essentially another toxic substance that your body must eliminate, and is therefore not recommended in this eating plan). And if you do drink coffee and tea, they simply cannot have cream and sugar, or even milk and honey for that matter.

Other calorie-containing drinks you must be sure to eliminate are alcohol of every kind, milk, and all fruit juices. Vegetable juices do not apply, and actually will count as whole food, which I will elaborate on in a later section.

10. Control Your Portions

While it isn't necessary to count every last calorie and gram of food you eat, it is important to control your portions. No matter how "clean" your diet is, even if you are eating nothing but healthy foods, if you eat too much of them, you will still gain weight. It all boils down to calories in and calories out. If you burn more calories than you eat, you will lose weight. If you consume more calories than you burn, you will gain weight, period.

Portion control is not hard; again, you just need to use your common sense. For example, under no circumstance should you ever go back for second helpings. Take a moderate amount of food the first time, and then leave it at that. If you are still hungry, don't worry; it won't be long before you will be eating again. Also, by waiting twenty minutes, you will find that your hunger usually vanishes. This is because hunger signals take a long time just to register in your brain. If you keep eating until you are full, you have actually *stuffed yourself.*

And while following the "Ten Nutritional Commandments" can propel you into an incredible total body transformation and help you get sexy and sculpted arms in record time, if you ignore proper portion control, you will simply spin your wheels and be frustrated with your lack of results.

This won't take much effort on your part, however, as I have devised a method to make it supersimple for you. In the "Individual Meal Breakdown" section, I will lay out the correct portion sizes for everything you will be eating in your daily meals. For individuals who require more or fewer calories (based on your current weight), I will also show you how to modify the amounts of specific foods to suit your body, in "How to Adjust Your Portion Sizes."

Food Guidelines–What to Eat, What Not to Eat

In this section, I will lay out the details of what foods you should be eating and which ones you should avoid completely. I will also make suggestions for substitutions where appropriate: For example, instead of coffee, drink green tea, and instead of regular bread, switch to sprouted grain, no-flour bread. With the following food guidelines, you will then be able to select the foods that you prefer, and put them into your own personal nutrition plan by using the "Individual Meal Breakdown" section.

Liquids

You should be drinking ten glasses of water per day, minimum, and twelve are recommended. Drink nothing with calories in it, and nothing with artificial sweeteners. Drink lots of caffeine-free herbal tea, and replace your coffee with green tea.

I also recommend eliminating milk from your diet. Most people are at least *somewhat* lactose intolerant, and while they might not exhibit *obvious* physical symptoms, they can find it very difficult to eliminate any extra body fat until they take milk out of their diet. Lactose is a sugar, and in every cup of milk there are 12 grams of it, so it's best not to drink it at all. As for calcium, although milk does contain high amounts of it, it actually is not absorbed as well as other sources of calcium. For example, green leafy vegetables are a better, and more absorbable, source of calcium and should be staples in your diet.

To help you get enough fluid intake, I recommend keeping a measured water bottle with you at all times to keep track of how much you drink every day. For example, I often keep a 1-liter water bottle on my desk, and I make sure that I have downed the whole thing once before 11:00 a.m., another before 4:00 p.m., and one more before 9:00 p.m., to ensure a minimum of 3 liters per day.

A note on tea and coffee: Although I do recommend eliminating coffee and black tea from your diet for reasons explained in previous sections, I realize that this may take some time to do, especially if you have been consuming large amounts for many years. At the very least, you should reduce your consumption to two cups or less per day, and be sure that you aren't using any cream or sugar.

It should be noted that green tea *does* have caffeine, but because it also has so many health-promoting substances in it (high levels of antioxidants, for example), it really isn't necessary to limit the amount of green tea you drink. In fact, drinking a cup or two of green tea a day is something I highly recommend.

Include . . .

▶ Water (lots of it)

▶ Caffeine-free herbal tea

▶ Green tea (regular or decaffeinated)

Don't include (or limit where noted) . . .

▶ Coffee (one or two cups a day if impossible to give up)

▶ Black tea (one or two cups a day if impossible to give up)

▶ Artificially sweetened drinks

▶ Diet drinks

▶ Sodas (diet or otherwise)

▶ Milk

▶ Fruit juice

▶ Alcohol

Fruits and Veggies

One of the most important aspects of the Totally Toned Arms Nutrition Plan is that every meal must include at least one serving of veggies, and each of your first three meals of the day should contain fruit. You know by now the absolute necessity of these foods in order to provide you with the essential nutrition that many people sorely lack and to help you detoxify your body naturally. This will help you get the fat-burning and health-improving results you want.

With regard to eating veggies in the morning, some people find this difficult. If you have trouble eating vegetables at breakfast, consider picking up premade vegetable juice, such as V8 juice, or make your own with a juice extractor. There is no reason for vegetable juice to taste bad, and there are a number of great juicing books available that have recipes for making your own at home.

Note: Commandment 9, which instructs you to drink nothing with calories in it, *does not apply* to vegetable juice. This is because vegetable juice contains very few calories while still containing plenty of fiber, and it is absolutely stacked with nutrition. For these reasons, vegetable juice can be classified as a "whole food" rather than a drink. The same applies to freshly made smoothies, which are a great way to get fruit, veggies, and lean protein in a quick and tasty way. Although they are liquid, they will still be classified as a meal. Therefore, vegetable juice and smoothies should not be counted toward your daily fluid intake, either.

Include . . .

- ▶ All vegetables (e.g., broccoli, spinach, carrots, beets, cauliflower, etc.)
- ▶ All fruits (e.g., apples, pears, oranges, grapefruits, pomegranates, etc.)

Don't include (or limit where noted) . . .

- ▶ None

The following are typically thought of as vegetables, but in this program I am classifying them as a starch:

- ▶ Peas (shelled, frozen, or raw)
- ▶ Corn (on the cob, fresh, or frozen)
- ▶ Potatoes
- ▶ Sweet potatoes
- ▶ Yams

This does *not* mean that these foods should be eliminated, but simply that different rules apply to them. For the purposes of this program, they are *not* vegetables. See the "Carbohydrates/Starches" section for more information.

Protein

Next to fruit and veggies, lean protein should be the cornerstone of every single meal. Most women would do well to ensure that they get, at the very least, 100 grams of protein a day. This can be accomplished by ensuring you get an average serving size of protein at each of your six daily meals. Eggs, fish, lamb, lean beef, and light poultry meat are all perfect examples of lean protein. But don't forget that nuts and seeds, beans and legumes, low-fat cottage cheese, and protein powders all fit in here as well; it doesn't have to be meat to be protein. It is also typically thought that red meat is a bad source of protein, but this is not entirely true. By selecting cuts of beef that are *lean* and trimming away any visible fat before cooking, you are actually getting a very lean source of protein, which is perfectly acceptable and well suited to a healthy eating plan.

Include . . .

▶ Lean cuts of beef

▶ All fish and shellfish (even high-fat fish such as salmon)

▶ Lean cuts of lamb

▶ White poultry meat (dark is very high in fat)

▶ Lean cuts of pork

▶ Eggs (whole or egg whites)

▶ Nuts and seeds

▶ Beans and legumes

▶ Low-fat cottage cheese or skim mozzarella (limited portions only)

▶ Whey protein powder

Don't include . . .

▶ High-fat cuts of pork, beef, and lamb

▶ Highly salted and processed meats such as salami, various "loaves," pepperoni, bacon, etc. (Choose instead low-fat cuts of ham, chicken, turkey, or roast beef from the deli.)

▶ High-fat cheeses (Low-fat cottage cheese and skim mozzarella are good alternatives.)

▶ Dark poultry meat (Light meat without the skin is very low fat and a great alternative.)

Carbohydrates/Starches

While fruits and veggies provide carbohydrates in your diet, relatively speaking the vast majority of your carbs will be coming from starches and whole grains. And while they can be an important part of your diet, you must be absolutely certain to exercise strict portion control when it comes to this category. Nearly every one of the clients I've ever counseled on losing body fat, initially ate far too many foods from this category, and in portions that were nearly *double* what they needed. Starches, which include items such as potatoes, rice, pastas, breads, flour products, and even corn and peas, are all very energy-dense, carbohydrate-rich foods.

You will see in the later "Individual Meal Breakdown" section, where I teach you how to plan out your daily meals, that you will be consuming your starches *before* three in the afternoon. This way, you will provide yourself with all the slow-burning carbohydrates you need to power yourself through the day, *without overloading* at the end of the day with extra energy that won't be used. Unless you are highly active, such as an athlete or someone who works a very physical job, you simply do not need any more carbohydrate and starch past your lunchtime meal.

When it comes to making selections for the best whole grains to include in your diet, sources such as brown or wild rice, slow-cooking oats, sprouted grain breads (the no-flour variety), and ancient grains such as quinoa and spelt are all excellent choices. All these selections provide plenty of carbohydrates, fiber, protein, and many essential vitamins and minerals, yet they burn slowly and don't cause a spike in blood sugar like their processed and refined counterparts.

I am often met with hesitation when I make these recommendations for substantially cutting back on carbohydrate consumption. As a society, we have become completely ingrained (no pun intended) with the idea that each meal should have a large helping of potato, pasta, or rice. However, the vast majority of us work at desk jobs or occupations where we stand or sit in one spot *all day long*. Most of us aren't farming, or logging, or mining anymore. We simply *do not have the same energy requirements* that the lifestyles of a hundred years ago did, and if we continue to eat the amount of carbohydrates that we have been, we are only going to keep getting fatter.

Remember, what isn't used is stored. And while *some* carbohydrates are essential, you must keep this amount in check. If you are eating adequate fruits and veggies, as I recommend, then you are probably getting all the carbohydrates you need from that alone. Therefore, you don't *have* to include additional carbs. Of course, for most people, this is too big of a step to take at first, so that is why

I recommend cutting out your starch intake after your noon meal, ensuring that any additional carbs you eat throughout the rest of the day will only come from vegetable sources. This will help safeguard you from overconsuming additional carbohydrates that, in all likelihood, would *not* be burned up, and instead make their way to additional body fat stores.

Include . . .

▸ Slow-cooking, "old-fashioned" or large-flake oats

▸ Brown or wild rice

▸ Corn (may be eliminated for even better results)

▸ Peas

▸ Quinoa

▸ Spelt

▸ Amaranth

▸ Sprouted grain breads and wraps (the no-flour variety)

▸ Yams

▸ Sweet potatoes

▸ Turnips

▸ Potatoes (may be eliminated for even better results)

Don't include . . .

▸ Noodles (rice, egg, or otherwise)

▸ Instant oats or packaged oatmeal

▸ White rice

▸   Pasta (whole wheat, rice, or regular)

▸   Flour products (breads, cakes, cookies, pastries, etc.)

▸   Sugar, honey, corn syrup, brown sugar

Fats

Fats get a bad rap, but it's more a case of mistaken identity than anything. As is often the case, the vast majority of North Americans eat far too much saturated fat, and far too little unsaturated fat. Fat is an absolute necessity to a healthy body and is needed to help you burn off extra body fat, but you need to be selective about the *type* of fat that you are consuming.

Most of your protein sources are going to have at least a little fat in them, so you will be getting some of what you need from these sources. Nuts and seeds have a lot of it (however, this is of the healthy variety). And while some people like to supplement their diets with healthy oils such as flaxseed oil or fish oil, it isn't entirely necessary if you are eating a well-varied diet that includes lots of fish, nuts, seeds, and olive oil.

As long as you stick to the healthy unsaturated oils when cooking and be sure to avoid large amounts of saturated fats, then that is all the thought you will need to give to the fat content of your diet.

Note: Trans fats should be eliminated completely. There are far too many health risks associated with these man-made fats, and they have no place in a healthy eating plan.

Include . . .

▶ Unsaturated oils: flaxseed, olive, canola, sesame, fish, etc.

▶ Nonhydrogenated margarines

Don't include . . .

▶ Butter

▶ Lard

▶ Hydrogenated oils and trans fats (Often used in many margarines—check the label! Trans fats are also common in commercially prepared cakes, cookies, pies, etc.)

▶ Large amounts of animal fats (These can be avoided by eating skinless poultry, trimming all excess visible fat from your cuts of meat, and choosing leaner cuts to begin with.)

Individual Meal Breakdown

Now that you have a good understanding of the "Ten Nutritional Commandments" and the types of foods that you should and should not be eating, it's time to put this all together into a workable plan that you can follow day to day.

What I will be doing in this section is taking you through what you should be eating for each of your daily six meals. I will outline specific serving sizes for each of the components that need to be included in the meal, and then you will be able to select what specific foods you want to eat based on the guidelines in the previous section. To help give you some ideas of what to eat, in the section that follows, I will provide you with some sample meal plans that you can use to get started.

As for specific meal timing, for each meal I will give you the general time that you should be eating. With regards to your workouts, it is best to eat no sooner than an hour before you work out. However, you can, and should, eat as soon after your workout as possible. Nutrient timing is a very complex subject in itself, but basically speaking, if you just keep your meals evenly distributed throughout the day, you will get great results and don't need to think about it any more than that.

Note: The following recommendations are for a woman weighing between 140 and 160 pounds and following the exercise program listed in this book. Your individual body weight and activity levels alter your nutritional requirements substantially. For instructions on how to modify the amounts of food in the following meals to suit your current weight, please see "How to Adjust Your Portion Sizes."

You will notice that I do not include beverages in the "Individual Meal Breakdown." This is because I expect you to be drinking water throughout the day, not just at mealtimes. Remember that ten to twelve glasses are the minimum.

Meal 1—Breakfast

Breakfast really is the most important meal of the day. Done correctly, a good breakfast can rev up your metabolism first thing in the morning and keep it burning all day long. It will start the ever-important rebuilding process from your previous day's workout, give you a boost of energy, and fuel you properly so you make it through your entire day without ever feeling drained or sluggish. Unfortunately, many people set themselves up for failure first thing in the morning by eating an improper breakfast, or skipping it all together.

Because we're all so busy in the morning and just trying to get out the door on time, breakfast is easy to forget. In fact, many people I've worked with don't really have much of an appetite in the morning (a sure sign of a slow metabolism) and therefore don't eat anything until they've been up and about for a few hours.

Breakfast's purpose is to give you a kick-start of quick energy, plus some slow-burning energy to last throughout the day. It also needs to provide plenty of protein to start the rebuilding process from the previous day's workout.

If you don't have time to cook breakfast, then a smoothie is your best option here. You can throw everything into a blender, give it a quick spin, and you are out the door in less than a few minutes. This is also a great way to "hide" veggies if you are uncomfortable with the idea of eating them at breakfast: Just toss some spinach, beet tops, and carrots into your smoothie, and with the addition of some fresh fruit, you won't even know they are there.

Note: As another option for getting veggies in the morning, you could also use a scoop of a commercially prepared "greens" product instead. These powders, while not as *ideal* as fresh veggies, are an appropriate substitute and can be added to any smoothie to get those veggies in when you otherwise wouldn't be able to. Just be sure that you substitute a greens product for veggies in only *one meal a day*.

Build Your Breakfast

1 serving of whole grains

(quick or slow-cooking oats, sprouted grain bread, quinoa, oat bran, etc.)

1 serving of fruit

(mixed berries, apple, banana, pear, etc.)

1 serving of vegetables

(sliced peppers, broccoli, spinach, greens powder, etc.)

1 serving of lean protein

(eggs and egg whites, lean animal protein, protein powder, etc.)

1 serving of healthy fat

(olive, flaxseed, or fish oil, nonhydrogenated light margarine, egg yolk, etc.)

Meal 2–Midmorning Snack

The midmorning snack should be eaten no more than 2 or 3 hours after breakfast. The primary goal of this meal is to give you some sustained fuel without overloading on carbs, which will cause a blood sugar crash later. A little protein is also necessary to keep your metabolism burning and to keep the rebuilding process going seamlessly. The addition of some healthy fat at this time helps to slow digestion and keep hunger at bay until your next meal.

Build Your Midmorning Snack

1 serving of fruit

1 serving of vegetables

½ serving of lean protein

1 serving of healthy fat

Meal 3—Lunch

Lunch should follow the midmorning snack by no more than 2 or 3 hours, and should be the next largest meal of the day. Here you want to include a larger serving of protein, with your usual serving of vegetables, and a medium serving of carbohydrate in the form of whole grains. You should also include a piece of fresh fruit with this meal to give you the energy you need for your workout. If you work out *before noon*, the fruit will help replenish your energy stores. If you work out *after noon*, the fruit will ensure that you are "topped up" with the quick burst of energy you will need for your exercise session. To avoid the midafternoon crash, you will want to make sure that you do not go overboard with the rest of your carbs here, so pay attention to your portion sizes of whole grains.

Build Your Lunch

1 serving of lean protein

1 serving of vegetables

1 serving of fruit

1 serving of whole grains

1 small serving of healthy fat

Meal 4—Midafternoon Snack

The midafternoon snack should be about 3 hours after lunch (which for most people will land at around 3:00 p.m.) and is one of the most important, but often neglected, meals of the day. This is the meal that will allow you to get through your afternoon with energy to spare, and will keep hunger in check until dinnertime. This meal should not include any fruit or whole grains, as the day's carbohydrate requirements will have already been fulfilled by this time. Under no circumstances should you ever skip this meal, as doing so will set you up for failure later in the evening owing to rapidly decreasing blood sugar levels that will trigger extreme hunger.

Build Your Midafternoon Snack

1 serving of vegetables

½ serving lean protein

1 serving of healthy fat

Meal 5—Dinner

For most of us in North America, dinner is the largest meal of the day. In fact, in reviewing hundreds of my clients' personal nutritional journals, I have found that the average person eats nearly 75 *percent of their calories in the evening*!

This is completely *opposite* from the way we should eat. Since your metabolism slows down later in the day, as do your activity levels, all those calories you are consuming before you go to bed aren't getting used.

It's important to *completely restrict* the amount of carbohydrate you consume at this point in the day, relying solely on vegetables for any extra carbs you consume. Lean protein and healthy fats are important here to keep you feeling satisfied and to continue building lean muscle tissue as well, but there should be no fruit or whole grains consumed.

If you are really hungry at this point (which you shouldn't be if you've been following the meal plan properly), then load up on veggies. It is also a good idea to start each dinner with a large green salad to fill you up first.

Build Your Dinner

1–2 large servings of vegetables

1 serving of lean protein

1 serving of healthy fat

Meal 6—Evening Snack

While many trainers will insist that you should not eat anything after dinner, there is a way you can have a small bite to eat, and actually have it benefit you. As you sleep, you are still burning calories (albeit a much smaller number than during your waking hours), but more importantly, this is when your body shifts into repair and recovery mode.

If you provide your body with some protein before you go to sleep, and add to that a little healthy fat to slow the speed at which it is digested, you can allow your body to repair itself while you sleep, *without* risking the addition of any extra body fat. Extra attention must be paid to portion control at this time, as you must keep the total calorie content of this meal low, and under no circumstances should you be eating any carbs at this time unless they are in the form of vegetables.

Build Your Evening Snack

½ serving of lean protein

½ serving of healthy fat

½ serving of vegetables

Planning Your Own Meals

The great thing about the Totally Toned Arms Eating Plan is that you design it yourself based on what you like to eat, and you don't need to be a nutritionist or a trainer to figure it all out. The "Food Guidelines" tell you what you can and cannot eat, and the "Individual Meal Breakdown" shows you what each meal should comprise and in what portions.

Here is what a two-day meal plan *might* look like for a woman who currently weighs between 140 and 160 pounds. By no means must you copy these meals exactly; they are just suggestions to get you thinking about the options that you have. Remember, as long as you stick to the "Food Guidelines" and the "Individual Meal Breakdown," you can't go wrong. Use your imagination to try and get as much variety into your personal nutrition plan as possible.

Day 1

Breakfast

Smoothie blended with 1 cup mixed frozen berries, ½ cup oats, 1 scoop vanilla protein powder, 2 teaspoons flaxseed oil, 1 cup fresh vegetable juice, and water to reach desired consistency

Midmorning Snack

½ cup fat-free cottage cheese mixed with 2 tablespoons sliced almonds, 1 sliced apple, and celery and carrot sticks

Lunch

4 ounces fat-free tuna salad served on a slice of sprouted grain bread and a large green salad with 3 tablespoons of lemon juice and olive oil dressing; 1 medium orange for dessert

Midafternoon Snack

1 cup sliced fresh peppers, 3 slices low-fat turkey breast, and 1 ounce unsalted nuts

Dinner

1 medium grilled chicken breast and mixed greens salad with sliced peppers, carrots, and snap peas; serve with 3 tablespoons olive oil, lemon juice, and fresh garlic dressing

Evening Snack

2 large celery stalks topped with 1 tablespoon natural peanut butter

Day 2

Breakfast

Omelet made with 2 whole eggs, and 1 cup combined sliced peppers, onions, and mushrooms, and served on 1 slice sprouted grain toast; include 1 small or ½ large grapefruit

Midmorning Snack

½ cup fat-free plain yogurt mixed with 1 ounce sliced almonds and 1 cup fresh berries; serve with fresh chopped broccoli and cauliflower pieces

Lunch

Wrap made with 1 sprouted grain tortilla, 1 medium grilled chicken breast, 1 cup total of broccoli sprouts, sliced peppers, lettuce, and spinach, and dress with 2 tablespoons low-fat Italian dressing; serve with 1 medium apple for dessert

Midafternoon Snack

1 small can low-fat, ready-to-eat tuna salad, served on romaine lettuce leaves with raw celery and carrot sticks on the side

Dinner

4.5-ounce grilled salmon steak served on a large bed (at least 2 cups) of fresh spinach and mixed greens; drizzle with 2 tablespoons combined lemon juice and olive oil

Evening Snack

1 cup boiled fresh or frozen edamame (green soybeans in the pod), drizzled with 1 teaspoon olive oil and seasoned with a pinch of sea salt

How to Adjust Your Portion Sizes

Instead of giving you a strict and regimented menu plan that you cannot deviate from, I have designed the Totally Toned Arms Nutrition Program to be highly customizable. This program can be altered to suit any individual's food preferences within a basic set of guidelines. And while the freedom to make your own food choices, instead of me making them for you, should have you breathing a sigh of relief, there is one problem with this arrangement: portion control.

As I have mentioned already, while this nutrition program will have you making wonderful and healthy changes to your eating habits, it will all be for naught if proper adherence to portion control is not exercised. So how do we go about making this work for you personally?

The trick is adjusting the portions given in the "Individual Meal Breakdown" to fit your current body weight. The number of calories you burn in a day is greatly dictated by how much you weigh and how active you are. Since your general activity level is known (you will be doing the exercise program in this book), the only variable of concern is your body weight. In a moment, I will show you how to adjust the portion sizes in this manual to suit your *current* weight. But first, let me explain some important points on caloric requirements.

The number of calories your body needs will increase as your body weight increases, and decrease as you lose weight, but *only to a certain point*. There exist many equations that can help you determine how many calories your body needs, but these equations all have an inherent flaw: They put far too much emphasis on body weight, and not enough on actual lean body mass. For example, these equations would assume that if you weigh 250 pounds, you will be burning far more calories than a woman who weighs 200 pounds. In my experience, this is not the case.

For women, as body weight increases over and above 180 pounds, nearly all of the additional weight will be excess body fat and fluid, *not* muscle mass and lean tissue. It is important to remember that *only lean tissue is metabolically active* and requires calories to survive. Therefore, both a woman who is 180 pounds and one who is 200 pounds will have similar lean tissue mass, but it will be their body fat and fluid levels that differ. This means that, in actuality, they both require about the same calories. The same is true for smaller women. There is a bottom level for how many calories you need for proper functioning, and no woman should drop below this.

The reason I mention all of this is because if you are over and above a certain body weight, and you try to calculate how many calories you need, you could very well end up gaining weight owing to a massive overestimation of your nutritional needs. For lighter women, you run the risk of becoming malnourished if you cut your calories too far.

However, there is no need to become overly concerned, because I am going to keep things simple for you. All you need to do is refer to the list on page 122 to find out which weight category you fit into, and then adjust your portion sizes accordingly. Remember to revisit this chart from time to time. As you lose weight, you may find yourself dropping into a lower category, and thus you will need to readjust your portion sizes.

Portion Sizes Based on Body Weight

The following portion adjustments are based on the serving sizes listed on pages 124–125. The portion sizes in the two-day sample meal plans are intended for a woman weighing between 140 and 160 pounds who is following the exercise program given in this book.

Less than 140 pounds: Reduce all portion sizes by ¼.

140 to 160 pounds: Keep all portion sizes the same.

Above 160 pounds: Increase all portion sizes by ¼.

Therefore, if you currently weigh 180 pounds, then the chart above instructs you to increase your portion sizes by ¼. This means that you will increase the portion size of *everything included in each meal by ¼* (see "Measuring Serving Sizes" for more info). If we take a look at the "Individual Meal Breakdown" for breakfast, we see the following:

1 serving of whole grains
   (*quick or slow-cooking oats, sprouted grain bread, quinoa, oat bran, etc.*)

1 serving of fruit
   (*berries, apple, banana, pear, etc.*)

1 serving of vegetables
   (*sliced peppers, broccoli, spinach, greens powder, etc.*)

1 serving of lean protein
   (*eggs and egg whites, lean animal protein, protein powder, etc.*)

1 serving of healthy fat
   (*olive, flaxseed, or fish oil, nonhydrogenated light margarine, etc.*)

After increasing everything in this meal by ¼, this is what your breakfast would look like:

1 ¼ servings of whole grains

(*quick or slow-cooking oats, sprouted grain bread, quinoa, oat bran, etc.*)

1 ¼ servings of fruit

(*berries, apple, banana, pear, etc.*)

1 ¼ servings of vegetables

(*sliced peppers, broccoli, spinach, greens powder, etc.*)

1 ¼ servings of lean protein

(*eggs and egg whites, lean animal protein, protein powder, etc.*)

1 ¼ servings of healthy fat

(*olive, flaxseed, or fish oil, nonhydrogenated light margarine, etc.*)

For a woman who is eating a lot of junk food, not exercising, and following other unhealthy habits, counting calories becomes far more important. This is because her body will be primed for fat storage, and her metabolism will be low. In your case, you will be burning lots of calories through exercise, and your metabolism will be high. A little extra *healthy* food will be burned up, or used to repair your muscles from your workout; therefore, you don't need to be exact down to the gram and calorie.

Measuring Serving Sizes

Serving sizes can vary quite significantly, depending on the nutritional organization that publishes them. For instance, there are some discrepancies between Canadian, American, and European nutritional authorities as to what constitutes one serving of carbohydrates.

To keep things simple, you will be using the serving sizes given *below* and can ignore the others. These will help you measure out your portions perfectly, and keep you on track with the Totally Toned Arms Nutrition Program.

Liquids

1 serving = 1 cup or 8 ounces or 250 milliliters

Protein

1 serving = 4.5 ounces or 125 grams of meat or fish, or 2 whole eggs, or a 30-gram scoop of protein powder, or 1 ounce of nuts and seeds, or 1 cup of low-fat cottage cheese

Note: When using whole eggs and nuts and seeds, for every one serving of protein, *also* count one serving of fat.

Fats

1 serving = 2 teaspoons of oil or 2 teaspoons of margarine

Vegetables

1 serving = 1 cup of chopped fresh veggies, or 2 cups of mixed salad greens or spinach (because salad greens and spinach are less dense than other vegetables, you will require twice the volume), or one 15-gram scoop of greens powder

Note: For vegetables, the serving size given is actually a *minimum*. Feel free to eat *more* of this category if you wish, but be sure to get at least the serving recommended. Also, don't rely on powdered greens products for more than just a single meal each day.

Fruit

1 serving = 1 cup of berries, or 1 medium orange, apple, pear, grapefruit, etc.

Note: If you are required to reduce your fruit serving by ¼ to fit your portion size, then simply eat *half of a large piece of fruit*. If you need to increase the portion size by ¼, then *eat a large piece of fruit*. This way, you aren't trying to chop ¼ out of a whole piece of fruit.

Carbohydrates

1 serving = ½ cup of uncooked oats or ½ cup of uncooked rice or 1 slice of sprouted grain bread, or 1 sprouted grain tortilla, or 1 medium potato or sweet potato, or 1 cup of corn or peas, or 1 corn on the cob

Grocery Checklist

Below is a list of the staple foods that you should have in your pantry and fridge before you start the Totally Toned Arms Nutrition Program. These are merely suggestions to get you started. It is highly recommended that you sit down once each week and plan out each of your weekly meals, making a grocery list as you go. You will then only have to do your grocery shopping once a week, and you will never be stuck in front of the fridge wondering what to eat.

Dairy Section and Cold Case Items

Fat-free cottage cheese

Nonhydrogenated margarine

Plain 1% yogurt

Skim mozzarella cheese

Deli and Meat Department

Boneless, skinless chicken breasts

Low-fat sliced turkey or chicken breast

Wild salmon, cod, or snapper fillets

Produce Section

Broccoli

Carrots

Celery

Green and red bell peppers

Lemons and limes (combine with olive oil for salad dressings)

Medium- or small-sized pink grapefruits

Medium-sized apples

Prewashed mixed green salad

Prewashed spinach

Dry and Canned Goods

Extra-virgin olive oil

Green tea

Large-flake or "old-fashioned" oats

Sprouted grain bread

Sprouted grain tortillas

Tuna canned in water

Supplements

Powdered greens

Whey protein powder (vanilla is best)

The 21-Day Program

THE TOTALLY TONED ARMS TRAINING PROGRAM combines both an interval-style cardiovascular training program with a circuit-format strength training program. The workout program is broken down into four separate phases, which are as follows:

▸ Quick Start Phase (7 days)

▸ Level 1 Phase (7 days)

▸ Level 2 Phase (7 days)

▸ Maintenance Phase (Beyond 21 days)

Cardiovascular Training Instructions

Choose one of the exercises from the following list for your daily cardiovascular exercise (refer to "Cardiovascular Training" for more details on choosing an appropriate cardio exercise):

▸ Elliptical/cross-trainer

▸ Walking/jogging/running—treadmill, road, or trail

▸ Rowing—actual or machine simulated

▸ Skipping

▸ Shadowboxing

▸ Swimming

You do not always have to choose the same exercise, so feel free to pick and choose from this list to add variety to your workouts, but you must select one option from *this* list.

Be sure to have your heart rate intensities already calculated, as described in "Cardiovascular Training," if you will be using a heart rate monitor.

If you will be using perceived exertion to monitor your intensity rate, then it is recommended that you review the different ratings as they relate to specific intensity levels.

You will always start each workout with your cardiovascular exercise, and you will also begin with a warm-up of 2 minutes. The goal of the warm-up is to bring your heart rate up, get you warm, and hopefully have you just starting to break a sweat.

Immediately after you complete the warm-up, you will start your first high-intensity interval for the given time. Once you complete your high-intensity interval, you will follow this with the low-intensity interval for its given time. You will then repeat this cycle of high intensity and low intensity for the number of sets.

Every week you will be making adjustments to the interval durations, so it is important to pay close attention to these in your daily instruction.

Strength Training Instructions

Circuit

The strength training exercises are to be done as a circuit. This means you will start with the first exercise listed, then immediately go to the next, and then the next, etc., without stopping to rest. Completing every exercise on the list counts as a single set. You will then stop to rest for the listed rest time. The whole series of exercises is then repeated for the number of sets given.

Reps

For each exercise you will be given a number of repetitions, or "reps," that you are required to lift the weight. Be sure to use a weight that is heavy enough that it causes temporary failure for each set, but is not too heavy that you cannot meet the minimum reps. You may find that in successive sets, you might have to lower the weight to achieve the proper repetitions. This is normal and is a result of the progressive fatigue that accumulates throughout the workout.

Note: During the first week of the program, the Quick Start Phase, you will not be taking each set to temporary failure. During this phase you will be performing the same workout, each day, for 7 days. You will not be taking a day off. This is done in order to adapt your body quickly and so you can start getting results right away. For this phase, you will see that you start at 6 reps, and each day you will add one rep until you have achieved 12 by the end of the week. **For this phase, and this phase only,** *if you feel that you can do more reps than what is listed, do not.* It is okay to do slightly *less* than you can handle because by the end of the week it will become much more challenging.

Many people start a training program and push themselves far too hard on the first few days before they know what their body can handle. This usually results in intense muscle soreness that leaves them unable to continue the program. However, by doing the same workout every day for 7 days and slowly building up the number of reps you perform, you ease yourself into the program and allow your body to adjust accordingly.

Active Rest

Active rest days are days in which you will not be performing interval cardio or strength training exercises. The term *active rest* is used to signify that you should still be moderately active, but not at an intensity that you would classify as a *workout*. For instance, during active rest days, it is recommended that you still walk for 20 to 30 minutes, or play a sport that you like. The goal here is to keep the body moving and burning calories, but at an intensity that is low enough that the body can still adequately recover from your workouts. It is completely up to you what you decide to do for your active rest. Just make it fun and enjoyable.

Day 1

Cardiovascular Training

WARM-UP

2 minutes

INTERVALS

High-intensity interval: 3 minutes at 75% or higher

Low-intensity interval: 3 minutes at 60% or lower

Sets: 3

Strength Training Circuit

Number of circuits: 3

Rest interval at end of circuit: 2 minutes

EXERCISE	REPETITIONS
A. Bench dips	6

| B. Burpees | 6 |

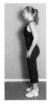 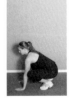 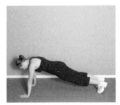

C. Jackknife 6

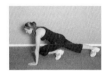 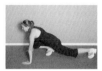

D. Mountain climbers 6

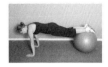

E. Bench push-ups 6

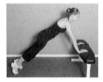 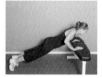

Day 2

Cardiovascular Training

WARM-UP

2 minutes

INTERVALS

High-intensity interval: 3 minutes at 75% or higher

Low-intensity interval: 3 minutes at 60% or lower

Sets: 3

Strength Training Circuit

Number of circuits: 3

Rest interval at end of circuit: 2 minutes

EXERCISE	REPETITIONS
A. Bench dips	7

B. Burpees	7

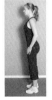 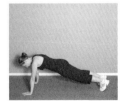

C. Jackknife 7

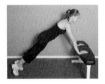

D. Mountain climbers 7

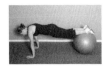 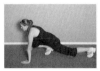

E. Bench push-ups 7

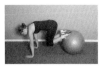 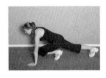

Day 3

Cardiovascular Training

WARM-UP

2 minutes

INTERVALS

High-intensity interval: 3 minutes at 75% or higher

Low-intensity interval: 3 minutes at 60% or lower

Sets: 3

Strength Training Circuit

Number of circuits: 3

Rest interval at end of circuit: 2 minutes

EXERCISE	REPETITIONS
A. Bench dips	8

B. Burpees	8

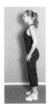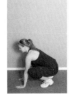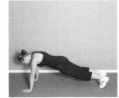

C. Jackknife   8

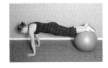

D. Mountain climbers   8

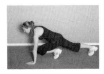 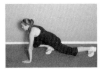

E. Bench push-ups   8

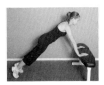

Day 4

Cardiovascular Training

WARM-UP

2 minutes

INTERVALS

High-intensity interval: 3 minutes at 75% or higher

Low-intensity interval: 3 minutes at 60% or lower

Sets: 3

Strength Training Circuit

Number of circuits: 3

Rest interval at end of circuit: 2 minutes

EXERCISE	REPETITIONS
A. Bench dips	9

B. Burpees	9

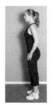 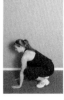 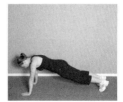

C. Jackknife 9

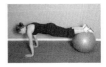 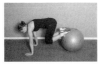

D. Mountain climbers 9

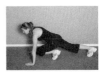 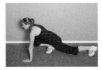

E. Bench push-ups 9

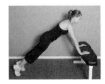 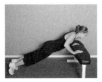

Day 5

Cardiovascular Training

WARM-UP

2 minutes

INTERVALS

High-intensity interval: 3 minutes at 75% or higher

Low-intensity interval: 3 minutes at 60% or lower

Sets: 3

Strength Training Circuit

Number of circuits: 3

Rest interval at end of circuit: 2 minutes

EXERCISE	REPETITIONS
A. Bench dips	10

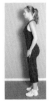

B. Burpees	10

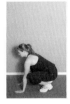 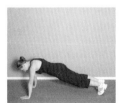

C. Jackknife 10

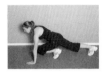 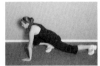

D. Mountain climbers 10

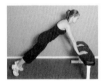 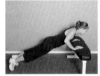

E. Bench push-ups 10

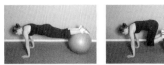

Day 6

Cardiovascular Training

WARM-UP

2 minutes

INTERVALS

High-intensity interval: 3 minutes at 75% or higher

Low-intensity interval: 3 minutes at 60% or lower

Sets: 3

Strength Training Circuit

Number of circuits: 3

Rest interval at end of circuit: 2 minutes

EXERCISE	REPETITIONS
A. Bench dips	11

B. Burpees	11

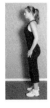 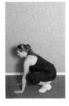 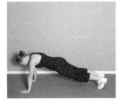

C. Jackknife   11

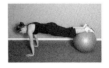

D. Mountain climbers   11

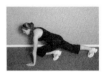 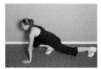

E. Bench push-ups   11

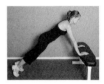 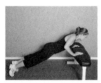

Day 7

Cardiovascular Training

WARM-UP

2 minutes

INTERVALS

High-intensity interval: 3 minutes at 70% or higher

Low-intensity interval: 3 minutes at 60% or lower

Sets: 3

Strength Training Circuit

Number of circuits: 3

Rest interval at end of circuit: 2 minutes

EXERCISE	REPETITIONS
A. Bench dips	12

B. Burpees	12

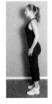 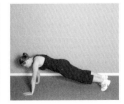

C. Jackknife   12

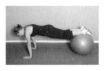

D. Mountain climbers   12

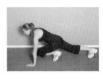 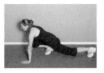

E. Bench push-ups   12

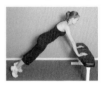 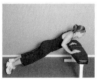

Day 8

Cardiovascular Training

WARM-UP

2 minutes

INTERVALS

High-intensity interval: 2 minutes at 80% or higher

Low-intensity interval: 2 minutes at 60% or lower

Sets: 4

Strength Training Circuit

Number of circuits: 3

Rest interval at end of circuit: 2 minutes

EXERCISE	REPETITIONS
A. Get-ups	6–8

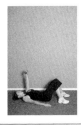 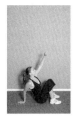 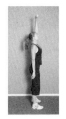

EXERCISE	REPETITIONS
B. Sumo squat and shoulder press	6–8

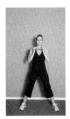 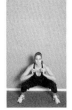 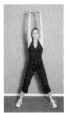

C. Lat pull-down 6–8

(HOME VERSION) (GYM VERSION)

  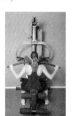 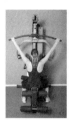

D. Chest press 6–8

(HOME VERSION) (GYM VERSION)

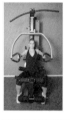 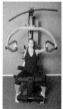

E. Weighted step-ups 6–8

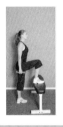 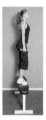

F. Upward crunch 6–8

Day 9

Cardiovascular Training

WARM-UP

2 minutes

INTERVALS

High-intensity interval: 2 minutes at 80% or higher

Low-intensity interval: 2 minutes at 60% or lower

Sets: 4

Strength Training Circuit

Number of circuits: 3

Rest interval at end of circuit: 2 minutes

EXERCISE	REPETITIONS
A. Single-leg bench dips	6–8

B. Cable curl 21s	6–8

(HOME VERSION)   (GYM VERSION)

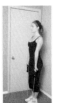 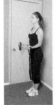 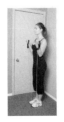 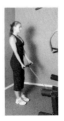 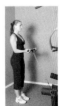 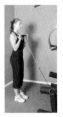

C. Chin-grip pull-down   6–8

(HOME VERSION)   (GYM VERSION)

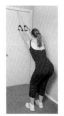 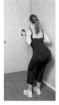 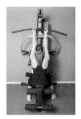 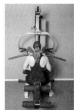

D. Dumbbell French press   6–8

(BENCH OPTION)   (FLOOR OPTION)

 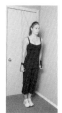

E. Band dips   6–8

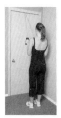 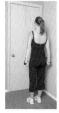

F. Triceps push-downs   6–8

(HOME VERSION)   (GYM VERSION)

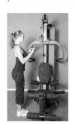 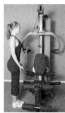

Day 10

Cardiovascular Training

WARM-UP

2 minutes

INTERVALS

High-intensity interval: 2 minutes at 80% or higher

Low-intensity interval: 2 minutes at 60% or lower

Sets: 4

Strength Training Circuit

Number of circuits: 3

Rest interval at end of circuit: 2 minutes

EXERCISE	REPETITIONS
A. Get-ups	8–10

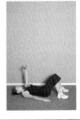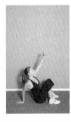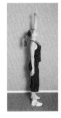

B. Sumo squat and shoulder press	8–10

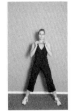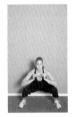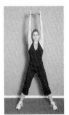

C. Lat pull-down   8–10

(HOME VERSION)   (GYM VERSION)

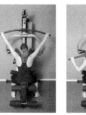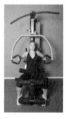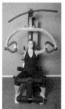

D. Chest press   8–10

(HOME VERSION)   (GYM VERSION)

E. Weighted step-ups   8–10

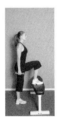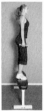

F. Upward crunch   8–10

Day 11

Cardiovascular Training

WARM-UP

2 minutes

INTERVALS

High-intensity interval: 2 minutes at 80% or higher

Low-intensity interval: 2 minutes at 60% or lower

Sets: 4

Strength Training Circuit

Number of circuits: 3

Rest interval at end of circuit: 2 minutes

EXERCISE	REPETITIONS
A. Single-leg bench dips	8–12

B. Cable curl 21s   8–12

(HOME VERSION)   (GYM VERSION)

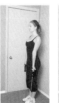 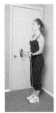 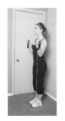 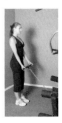 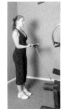 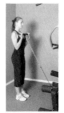

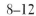

C. Chin-grip pull-down   8–12

(HOME VERSION)   (GYM VERSION)

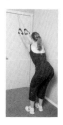 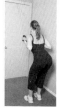 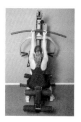 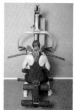

D. Dumbbell French press   8–12

(BENCH OPTION)   (FLOOR OPTION)

E. Band dips   8–12

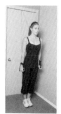

F. Triceps push-downs   8–12

(HOME VERSION)   (GYM VERSION)

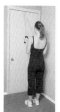 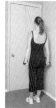 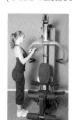 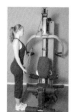

Day 12

Cardiovascular Training

WARM-UP

2 minutes

INTERVALS

High-intensity interval: 2 minutes at 80% or higher

Low-intensity interval: 2 minutes at 60% or lower

Sets: 4

Strength Training Circuit

Number of circuits: 3

Rest interval at end of circuit: 2 minutes

EXERCISE	REPETITIONS
A. Get-ups	10–12

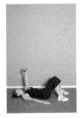 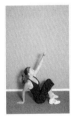 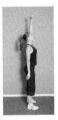

B. Sumo squat and shoulder press	10–12

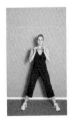 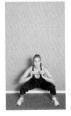 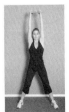

C. Lat pull-down 10–12

(HOME VERSION) (GYM VERSION)

 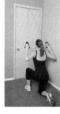 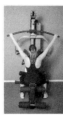 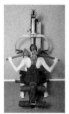

D. Chest press 10–12

(HOME VERSION) (GYM VERSION)

 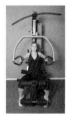 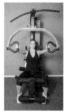

E. Weighted step-ups 10–12

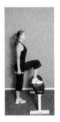 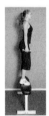

F. Upward crunch 10–12

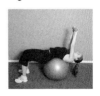

Days 13 and 14

Active rest only.

Day 15

Cardiovascular Training

WARM-UP

2 minutes

INTERVALS

High-intensity interval: 1 minute at 90% or higher

Low-intensity interval: 2 minutes at 60% or lower

Sets: 5

Strength Training Circuit

Number of circuits: 3

Rest interval at end of circuit: 2 minutes

EXERCISE	REPETITIONS
A. Dumbbell burpees	6–8

  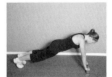

B. Clean and jerk   6–8

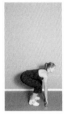 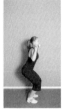 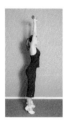

C. Seated cable rotation   6–8

(HOME VERSION)   (GYM VERSION)

 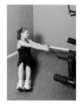 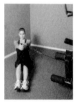

D. Kneeling chin-grip pull-down   6–8

(HOME VERSION)   (GYM VERSION)

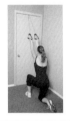 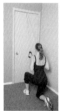 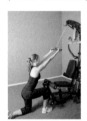 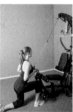

E. Toe tappers   6–8

F. Side-to-side push-ups   6–8

Day 16

Cardiovascular Training

WARM-UP

2 minutes

INTERVALS

High-intensity interval: 1 minute at 90% or higher

Low-intensity interval: 2 minutes at 60% or lower

Sets: 5

Strength Training Circuit

Number of circuits: 3

Rest interval at end of circuit: 2 minutes

EXERCISE	REPETITIONS
A. Bench and ball dip	6–8

(HOME VERSION)   (GYM VERSION)

B. One-arm preacher curl	6–8

(HOME VERSION)   (GYM VERSION)

 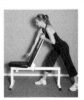

C. Twisting single-arm pull-down 6–8

(HOME VERSION) (GYM VERSION)

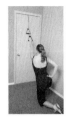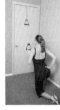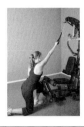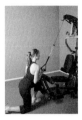

D. Narrow-width dumbbell press 6–8

(BENCH OPTION) (FLOOR OPTION)

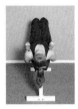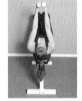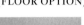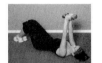

E. Slow-down push-ups 6–8

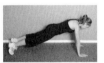

F. Reverse-grip dual-band pull-down and kickback 6–8

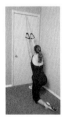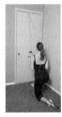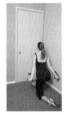

Day 17

Cardiovascular Training

WARM-UP

2 minutes

INTERVALS

High-intensity interval: 1 minute at 90% or higher

Low-intensity interval: 2 minutes at 60% or lower

Sets: 5

Strength Training Circuit

Number of circuits: 3

Rest interval at end of circuit: 2 minutes

EXERCISE	REPETITIONS
A. Dumbbell burpees	8–10

  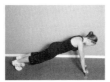

B. Clean and jerk	8–10

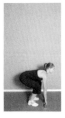 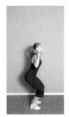 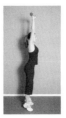

C. Seated cable rotation   8–10

(HOME VERSION)   (GYM VERSION)

 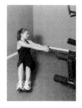 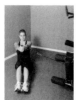

D. Kneeling chin-grip pull-down   8–10

(HOME VERSION)   (GYM VERSION)

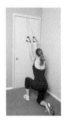 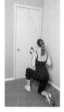 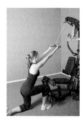 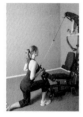 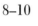

E. Toe tappers   8–10

F. Side-to-side push-ups   8–10

  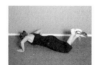

Day 18

Cardiovascular Training

WARM-UP

2 minutes

INTERVALS

High-intensity interval: 1 minute at 90% or higher

Low-intensity interval: 2 minutes at 60% or lower

Sets: 5

Strength Training Circuit

Number of circuits: 3

Rest interval at end of circuit: 2 minutes

EXERCISE	REPETITIONS
A. Bench and ball dip	8–12

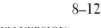

(HOME VERSION)   (GYM VERSION)

  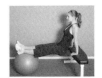

B. One-arm preacher curl   8–12

(HOME VERSION)   (GYM VERSION)

C. Twisting single-arm pull-down 8–12

(HOME VERSION) (GYM VERSION)

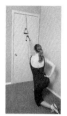 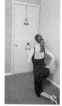 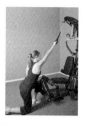 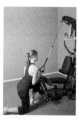

D. Narrow-width dumbbell press 8–12

(BENCH OPTION) (FLOOR OPTION)

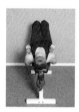 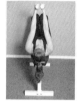

E. Slow-down push-ups 8–12

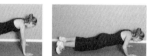

F. Reverse-grip dual-band pull-down and kickback 8–12

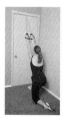 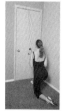 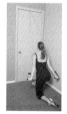

Day 19

Cardiovascular Training

WARM-UP

2 minutes

INTERVALS

High-intensity interval: 1 minute at 90% or higher

Low-intensity interval: 2 minutes at 60% or lower

Sets: 5

Strength Training Circuit

Number of circuits: 3

Rest interval at end of circuit: 2 minutes

EXERCISE	REPETITIONS
A. Dumbbell burpees	10–12

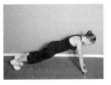

B. Clean and jerk	10–12

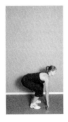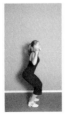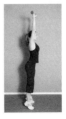

C. Seated cable rotation   10–12

(HOME VERSION)   (GYM VERSION)

 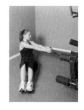

D. Kneeling chin-grip pull-down   10–12

(HOME VERSION)   (GYM VERSION)

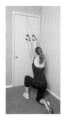 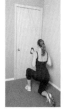 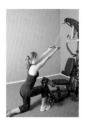 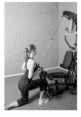

E. Toe tappers   10–12

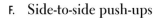

F. Side-to-side push-ups   10–12

   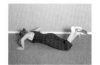

Days 20 and 21

Active rest.

The Maintenance Plan

TO MAINTAIN THE IMPROVEMENTS you've made to your body at this point, you won't need to work out as long or as often. It is necessary, however, to keep working the same muscle groups frequently enough so that they don't lose any of their tone or strength. You will also want to continue your cardiovascular work to keep your metabolism revving high and burning off extra calories.

You will now be doing three workouts per week, each separated by at least one day of active rest. The preferable schedule is to work out on Monday, Wednesday, and Friday. Each of the three workouts has a distinct goal: Workout 1 is a full-body workout that is designed to work all the major muscle groups. Workout 2 is a fat-burning workout designed to keep your metabolism burning hot and melt off any extra fat from your body. Workout 3 is an arm-sculpting workout used to further enhance the muscle definition and tone in your arms.

Maintenance Workout 1: Full Body (Monday)

Cardiovascular Training

WARM-UP

2 minutes

INTERVALS

High-intensity interval: 3 minutes at 75% or higher

Low-intensity interval: 2 minutes at 60% or lower

Sets: 3

Strength Training Circuit

Number of circuits: 3

Rest interval at end of circuit: 2 minutes

EXERCISE	REPETITIONS
A. Lat pull-down	8–12

(HOME VERSION)   (GYM VERSION)

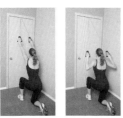 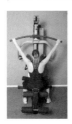 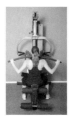

B. Chest press   8–12

(HOME VERSION)   (GYM VERSION)

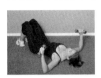 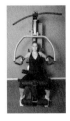 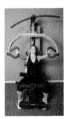

C. Sumo squat and shoulder press   8–12

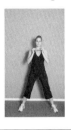 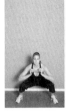 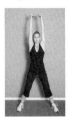

D. Upward crunch   8–12

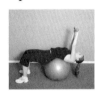

Maintenance Workout 2: Fat Burner (Wednesday)

Cardiovascular Training

WARM-UP

2 minutes

INTERVALS

High-intensity interval: 3 minutes at 75% or higher

Low-intensity interval: 2 minutes at 60% or lower

Sets: 3

Strength Training Circuit

Number of circuits: 3

Rest interval at end of circuit: 2 minutes

EXERCISE	REPETITIONS
A. Weighted step-ups	8–12

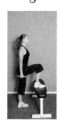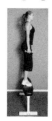

B. Clean and jerk   8–12

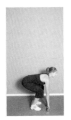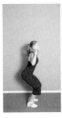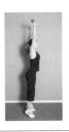

C. Side-to-side push-ups   8–12

D. Burpees   8–12

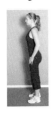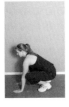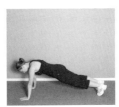

Maintenance Workout 3: Arm Sculpting (Friday)

Cardiovascular Training

WARM-UP

2 minutes

INTERVALS

High-intensity interval: 3 minutes at 75% or higher

Low-intensity interval: 2 minutes at 60% or lower

Sets: 3

Strength Training Circuit

Number of circuits: 3

Rest interval at end of circuit: 2 minutes

EXERCISE	REPETITIONS
A. Single-leg bench dips	8–12

B. Narrow-width dumbbell press 8–12

(BENCH OPTION) (FLOOR OPTION)

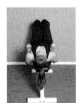 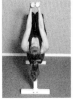

C. Band dips 8–12

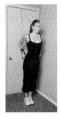 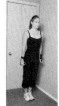

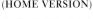

D. Triceps push-downs 8–12

(HOME VERSION) (GYM VERSION)

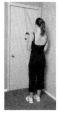 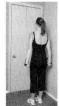 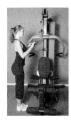 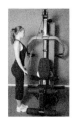

Tips for Maintaining Your Totally Toned Arms

▶ Remember the principle of progressive overload—in order to steadily improve, you must constantly overload and challenge your body. This doesn't always mean increasing weight. For example, one week you could increase all the weight you use by 5 percent, the following week you could increase the reps by 2, and the week after that you could reduce your rest intervals by 30 seconds. As long as you are changing and making it more difficult, your body will adapt and improve, and you will continue to get great results.

▶ Take a day off every now and again. If you feel that you are getting tired, rest for several days and don't exercise at all. The body is rebuilding only when you are resting, so it is important not to neglect your recovery.

▶ Pay attention to your nutrition plan. You don't need to make any changes to this aspect of the program to keep getting results, but nothing will ruin all your hard work faster than letting your healthy nutrition habits slip. Refer back to the "Ten Nutritional Commandments" every so often for a quick refresher on the main ideas.

▶ Read my blog. I post weekly hints and body-sculpting secrets, as well as new exercise ideas, nutritional help, and motivational tips at www.gosleevelessblog.com. You will even have access to new workout routines and you can also post your own questions and find out how to contact me personally.

▶ Commit to the maintenance plan. In order to keep your arms totally toned, it will take dedication to continued healthy eating and exercise.

ABOUT THE AUTHOR

TODAY, RYLAN IS A practicing kinesiologist, certified personal trainer, and certified strength and conditioning specialist. He owns and operates Adonis Fitness, a kinesiology practice and personal training studio, in Vernon, British Columbia. He is also the founder of GoSleeveless.com, and author of the Go Sleeveless e-book series.

Rylan lives with his wife, award-winning photographer, Ashley Duggan, in Coldstream, British Columbia, Canada.